PAIN MANAGEMENT - RESEARCH AND TECHNOLOGY

MANAGEMENT OF POSTOPERATIVE PAIN AFTER BARIATRIC SURGERY

PAIN MANAGEMENT - RESEARCH AND TECHNOLOGY

Additional books and e-books in this series can be found on Nova's website under the Series tab.

PAIN MANAGEMENT - RESEARCH AND TECHNOLOGY

MANAGEMENT OF POSTOPERATIVE PAIN AFTER BARIATRIC SURGERY

JAIME RUIZ-TOVAR
EDITOR

nova
Medicine & Health
New York

Library of Congress Cataloging-in-Publication Data

ISBN: 978-1-53614-284-6

Published by Nova Science Publishers, Inc. † New York

To Jaime, Mateo and Carolina,

the motors of my life.

CONTENTS

PREFACE

Obesity is actually considered a pandemia in developed countries. Some authors have even described it as the "pandemia of the 21st century". The reality is that obesity rates are increasing in Western countries and, even in developing countries, this begins to be a real problem.

Although we are living in a society based on the image of the person, based on the concept that a good image is associated with success (professional and personal success), obesity is not only an image problem, but it is a health problem. Obesity is associated with many metabolic disorders, such as diabetes mellitus, dyslipidemia, hypertension, sleep apnea-hypopnea syndrome, liver steatosis,... Far away from the psychological impact, obesity and its related comorbidities are silent diseases. These disorders are mostly asymptomatic and the patients do not complain of pain or any other symptom for many time, and it is just when the symptoms appear, that the damage is already irreversible. The objective of the fight against obesity is to prevent the appearance of these permanent damages, increasing then the life expectative and the quality of life.

The first step in the treatment of obesity is diet and physical activity, but the main problem is that the patients often tire from following both and abandon them, regaining the weight they have lost. After several attempts of diets with mild weight loss and regaining more and more weight, this situation leads to a morbidly obese status. The word "morbid" means that obesity itself represents a disease.

For morbidly obese patients, bariatric surgery is the best option to achieve a significant and maintained weight loss. The first bariatric procedures were performed 60 years ago as anecdotic procedures. Actually thousands of bariatric procedures are performed all around the world. Two facts have contributed to this exponential development of bariatric surgery. The first one is obviously the demand of the society. It is estimated that in Spain more than 1% of the population is morbidly obese and this rate will probably increase in the next decade, given the obesity rates in children and teenagers.

The second issue that has enormously contributed to the development of bariatric surgery is the laparoscopic technique. The first procedures performed by laparotomy, were associated with incredibly high complications and mortality rates. However, with the implementation of the laparoscopic approach world-wide, these complications rates have significantly decreased, implying that bariatric surgery is actually a safe procedure, with mortality rates under 0.5% and morbidity rates under 5%. Notwithstanding, the complications following laparoscopic bariatric techniques are still life-threatening conditions.

Despite minimally invasive surgery is the gold standard for bariatric surgery and most surgeries are performed by this approach, the surgical act itself is the same than in laparotomic surgery. However, one of the main advantages of laparoscopy is that the postoperative pain is significantly reduced, mainly because the parietal component of the pain (pain associated with the surgical incision) is decreased, due to 5-6 small incisions throughout the abdomen, in comparison with a 50cm long incision in laparotomies. Notwithstanding, minimally invasive approach does not imply absence of pain, as the small parietal incisions are associated with a certain feeling of pain, and the visceral component of the pain remains intact. Moreover, the CO_2 infusion in the peritoneal cavity also implies an irritation of the diaphragm, leading to the typical pain in the shoulder. Thus, a correct management of the postoperative pain is mandatory, in order to improve the patient´s recovery.

Bariatric surgery is actually amenable for following ERAS protocols. One of the main items of these ERAS protocols is the multimodal analgesia, consisting in the administration of different analgesic drugs by different ways, in order to reduce the pain sensation and the opioid needs. A correct analgesia does not necessarily imply the administration of analgesic agents, but there is increasing evidence in literature that other drugs might act on the inflammatory response after surgical damage and, modulating it, lead to a reduction in the pain feeling. I hope that this book, based on the current evidence of pain control methods can be helpful in the clinical practice. However, we must keep always in mine, that medical investigation obtains new data, drugs and approaches every day, so that current evidence can be outdated in the following decade, requiring future updates.

Finally, I want to thank to all the contributing authors, all of them friends and experts in the field of bariatric surgery, their availability, time and efforts to write all the chapters.

Jaime Ruiz-Tovar, MD, PhD
Editor

In: Management of Postoperative Pain … ISBN: 978-1-53614-284-6
Editor: Jaime Ruiz-Tovar

Chapter 1

PHYSIOPATHOLOGICAL BASIS OF POSTOPERATIVE PAIN

Dennis César Lévano-Linares[1,*], MD,
Patricia Sanchez-Salcedo[2],
Belen Manso Abajo[1], MD,
David Alías Jimenez[1], MD, PhD,
Manuel Durán Poveda[1], MD, PhD
and Jaime Ruíz-Tovar[1], MD, PhD

[1]Department of Surgery, University Hospital Rey Juan Carlos, Mostoles, Madrid, Spain
[2]Department of Surgical Nursery, Fundacion Jimenez Diaz, Madrid, Spain

ABSTRACT

The term "nociception" is derived from noci (*Latin word denoting damage or injury*) and is used to describe the neural response to traumatic or noxious stimuli. Nociceptive pain is produced by stimulation of specific sensitive receptors or nociceptors with variable density in tissues

[*] Corresponding Author: Dennis Cesar Levano-Linares, MD. Email: cesdenlinares@gmail.com.

such as skin, muscles, joints and viscera. Precisely the variation of the receptors density in tissues is which marks the sensory difference. The nociceptive nerve fibers are the Aδ and the C. The Aδ fibers are fast conducting myelinated activated by thermal, mechanothermic and high threshold mechanoreceptors. The C fibers are amylinic with slow conduction and a smaller field of receptivity. The majority of peripheral nociceptors present C fibers, and most of them are polymodal neurons, that is, they can react to mechanical, thermal or chemical stimuli. The postoperative pain (PP) is associated with a noxious stimulus wich is a component of injury and damage tissue with or without visceral involvement that sets in motion the mechanism of pain by activation of the called nociceptors. It is assumed that the intensity and character of the PP will vary with the surgical act and will cease with the healing of the tissues; however, some acute states may progress to chronicity. Showing a general outline, it can be stated that each sensory unit includes an organ-terminal receptor and a sensory fiber consisting of an accompanying axon, a dorsal root ganglion and a terminal axon in the spinal cord. In this chapter we will discuss the pathophysiological path of postoperative pain.

Keywords: nociceptive, postoperative pain

INTRODUCTION

Currently, we recognize that the etiology and treatment of pain produced by surgery is different than other clinical pain conditions like rheumatoid arthritis, fibromyalgia, or acute herpes zoster [1]. Many pain models may be useful for mechanistic studies but less valuable for developing novel targets to treat particular clinical pain conditions. In order to advance our treatment for acute PP, we must recognize, that many preclinical pain models, such as antigen-specific inflammation or receptor-specific, chemical stimuli (i.e., formalin or capsaicin), do not necessarily translate well to incisional pain mechanisms.

Theoretically, if the etiology and pathophysiology of the clinical condition are mimicked by the experimental model, analgesic target discovery may be improved. A second goal for preclinical rodent pain research is to make the endpoints for nociceptive testing have proximate translatability to clinical pain and analgesia [2]. Others have suggested that plasma levels of drugs for anti-nociception in animals and plasma concentrations for analgesia in human subjects be compared to improve the translatability of the models and the behavior in rodents. Limitations of pain models and behaviors may be one of several factors contributing to our limited success in developing new treatments for acute PP.

Because there has been a considerable debate regarding the clinical utility of rodent pain models, ourselves and others undertook studies on the etiology of nociception caused by incisions. Perhaps improving our understanding of the mechanisms for PP pain could increase the chances of developing new treatments for patients. Research on incisional pain mechanisms and relating these preclinical results to patient's symptoms has advanced our understanding of animal pain models, incision-induced pain-related behaviors in animal models, and PP mechanisms in patients. The long-term goal of PP research and acute incisional pain studies is for patients to undergo painless or nearly painless surgery.

1. Spontaneous Activity in Nociceptive Pathways after Incision

A key to translational pain research is to identity sensitized nociceptors and dorsal horn neurons that encode enhanced nociception so that targets transmitting these amplified signals can be evaluated for therapeutic potential. Ongoing or spontaneous activity (SA), one aspect of sensitization, is a stimulus-independent measurement of sensitization.

Characteristics of nociceptor sensitization after injury may include:

- spontaneous activity
- decreased response threshold
- increased response to a suprathreshold stimulus
- expansion of the receptive field
- an increase in the proportion of nociceptors responding to a particular stimulus [3].

We have undertaken a series of electrophysiologic studies in rats that had undergone plantar incision one day earlier and examined primary afferent and dorsal horn neuron activity and compared SA to unincised, sham operated animals. Most studies in our laboratory include not only measurements of ongoing SA but also, heat, mechanical and in some cases chemical sensitivity. SA is perhaps the most robust form of sensitization produced in postinjury states because no stimulus is required [4]. This review will focus on the generation of or an increase in the magnitude of SA of nociceptors and dorsal horn neurons produced by incisions.

One day after plantar incision, guarding behavior is usually significantly elevated [5]. We compared the SA of primary afferent nociceptors from rats that had undergone plantar incision [6] which included incision in skin, fascia and muscle one day earlier to those that had undergone sham operation. The nociceptors studied from the incision group innervated, at least in part, the area of the incision. Thirty-nine afferent fibers were recorded in the sham-operated group and 28 fibers were recorded in the plantar incision group on postoperative day 1, eleven of 28 nociceptors had SA in the incision group; the average frequency was approximately 17 imp/sec. In this study, the majority of spontaneously active Aδ and C-fibers' activity was greater than 15 imp/sec after incision. In the sham group, no afferents were spontaneously active. The origin of the SA was the incised tissue because local anesthetic infiltrated into the receptive field of the nociceptor in the hind-paw eliminated the activity [6]. It was surprising that the rate of SA was quite high in some nociceptive fibers.

We performed the corresponding experiment but this time recording dorsal horn neurons [7]. We measured behavior in rats that had undergone skin, fascia and muscle incision on postoperative day 1 and compared the behavior to rats that underwent a sham operation. The mean guarding pain scores were 15 and 0 in the incised and sham operated groups, respectively. Rats then underwent electrophysiology experiments, recordings of single dorsal horn neuron activity under general anesthesia. These dorsal horn neurons received input from afferent fibers innervating the glabrous skin of the hind-paw and had a mechanoreceptive field that again included at least part of the area of the incision. SA was identified in 9 of 27 neurons in the control group and 16 of 26 neurons in the incision group. The average dorsal horn SA in the incised rats was 19 imp/sec and was 10 imp/sec in the sham operated group. In this series, both the proportion of neurons with SA and the magnitude of SA were greater in the neurons from the incised group. Bupivacaine injection into the skin and deep tissue of the hind-paw reduced the level of SA in the incised group to the same level to that in the sham operated group [7]. Bupivacaine did not affect the magnitude of SA in the sham group. In summary, even though SA is intrinsic to some dorsal horn neurons, the proportion of neurons with SA and amount of SA were both increased one day after incision. Altogether, increased spinal dorsal horn neuron activity remained largely dependent on ongoing primary afferent input on postoperative day 1 when guarding behavior was evident. The SA was quite high in dorsal horn neurons and in agreement with the magnitude of activity in primary afferent nociceptors in similar groups of animals.

2. ANIMAL-EXPERIMENTAL RESEARCH

The original plantar incision model was developed in 1996 by Brennan et al. [4]. Briefly, under general anesthesia, a 1-cm longitudinal incision is performed through the glabrous skin, fascia, and plantar muscle of the rat hind paw. The skin is surgically sutured, then the animals recover from anesthesia; pain behavior can be measured from one hour thereafter. The combination of transsection of the skin, fascia, and retracted muscle compares well to the tissue trauma of patients undergoing surgery [8]. Similar to patients after surgery, rats develop short-lasting nonevoked guarding pain behavior (for a short time period of approximately 2 days after incision) and longer lasting evoked pain-related behavior to punctate mechanical stimuli (von Frey hairs); these pain behaviors are seen as a surrogate for nonevoked resting pain (lasting some days) and evoked pain (lasting several days till weeks) after surgery, respectively, and are therefore relevant to postoperative pain in patients [3]. Mechanical hyperalgesia occurs at the side of the incision (primary hyperalgesia) and in an area surrounding the injury (secondary hyperalgesia) for several days after the incision [9]. Furthermore, heat hyperalgesia, but not cold hyperalgesia [10], is prominent at the site of the incision lasting up to approximately 7 days [9]. Secondary heat hyperalgesia (usually measured as withdrawal thresholds to radiant heat) does not occur after this incision. Additionally, an incision model within the hairy skin hind paw of rats was developed for better investigation of secondary mechanical hyperalgesia in animals (gastrocnemius incision) [11]. More recently, anxiety- and depression-like behaviors were investigated after plantar incision; for example, rats show an increase in anxiety-like avoidance behaviors in the light/dark box and an increase in depression-like behavior (sucrose preference test) for some days after incision [12]. Other studies assessing anxiety-like behavior after incision in rats gave similar results by using slightly different approaches and study designs [13]. Interestingly, the anxiety-like behavior lasted longer than hyperalgesia in 2 (but not one) of these studies. As anxiety and other psychological factors such as depression, catastrophizing, and stress enhance acute and promote long-lasting pain after surgery, investigation of appropriate assays in animals might be relevant. In 2003, the rat plantar incision model has been transferred from the rat to the mouse with some modification (5 mm incision, one mattress suture, modulated assessment of mechanical, and heat hyperalgesia), with very similar results in behavioral experiments [14]. To investigate prolonged pain after a surgical incision more specifically, a skin and muscle retraction injury model (SMIR) was introduced. Here, a 1.5 to 2-cm incision is made in the skin of the medial inner thigh, 4 mm medial to the saphenous vein. The superficial (gracilis) muscle layer is then incised (7–10 mm) approximately 4 mm medial to the saphenous nerve and retracted with a microdissecting retractor for one hour. The tissue is sutured with silk. Mechanical hyperalgesia in the SMIR model lasts for up to 3 weeks and therefore much longer than after plantar incision, but heat hyperalgesia was not observed. Interestingly, the SMIR model has been transferred to a porcine model of prolonged incisional pain [15], which may have some very interesting advantages: For instance, pigs have a greater phylogenetic proximity with humans like a similar metabolism and a comparable skin anatomy with great homology in wound healing compared to rodents [16]. These advantages could be deployed for validating new topical and localized treatment options for postoperative, incisional pain in human. Many other pain models related to surgical and trauma injuries have been developed and a comprehensive overview can be found in the review quoted here [17]. One interesting model, for instance, is the back hairy skin incision model that represents another clinically relevant model for pain behavior after an incision in hairy skin [18]. However, because of space limitations and because of the fact that the plantar (and more recently the SMIR incision) is used most frequently for studying mechanisms of incisional pain, we will mainly focus on these 2 models. Finally, an incision model in humans is also available and may provide an important link between animal studies and patients.

3. Tissues Contributing to Guarding Pain and SA of Nociceptive Pathways

Three previous studies identified cutaneous nociceptors and examined SA before and after skin injury using scalpel blades or needles. In two separate studies, investigators used needles to penetrate the receptive fields of both Aδ and C fibers nociceptors recorded from cutaneous nerves in the cat [19, 20]. Activation during needle penetrations occurred and occasionally there were after discharges following the needle injury; however, no sustained SA was generated after the injury. Finally, Hammaleinin et al. recorded afferent fibers from the tibial nerve innervating the hindpaw of the rat hindpaw [21]. Activity was generated during incision and other forms of sensitization were evident; yet, no nociceptors developed ongoing, sustained SA after incision. It was surprising that nociceptors could not be activated immediately after incision because dorsal horn neurons generate some sustained SA during and after the same incisions. [22]. Dorsal horn neurons receive convergent input from a variety of tissues whereas nociceptors innervate specific tissues. Perhaps by selecting cutaneous nociceptors and incising their receptive fields, these cutaneous nociceptors did not generate SA after incision. We hypothesized that deep tissue incision that included fascia and muscle would generate SA in nociceptive pathways and produce unprovoked guarding pain but a skin only incision would not. We undertook a series of experiments incising skin only, skin, fascia and muscle (deep tissue) or sham (no operation) surgery. Guarding behavior was measured in separate groups of rats after sham, skin, or skin plus deep tissue incision 1 day later. A fourth group was studied 7 days after skin plus deep tissue incision when pain behaviors generally resolve. These same groups then underwent in vivo recording of single fiber nociceptors innervating the area of the incision. Compared with the sham control group, skin incision induced a small amount of guarding on the day of incision only, whereas skin plus deep tissue incision caused guarding for 5 days after incision and this behavior completely resolved on postoperative day 7 [23]. On postoperative day 1, skin incision (18%) produced a similar prevalence of SA in nociceptors as the sham operated group (13%), whereas skin plus deep tissue incision generated a greater prevalence of SA in nociceptors (61%); the rate of SA also tended to be greater after skin plus deep tissue incision (10 ± 3 imp/sec) versus the control group (6 ± 6) and skin incision group (6 ± 3 imp/sec). Seven days after skin plus deep tissue incision, when pain behaviors had resolved, the prevalence of SA (14%) and the amount of SA (0.3 ± 0.1) were similar as the sham group [24]. Incision of skin was not sufficient to produce guarding pain behavior but incision that included skin fascia and muscle was sufficient. In addition, skin incision was sufficient to produce the typical reduced heat withdrawal latency and reduced mechanical withdrawal threshold on postoperative day 1. An comparable series of experiments in four similar groups of rats was undertaken except in these four groups, dorsal horn neurons were recorded on postoperative day 1. Pain behaviors again demonstrated the importance of deep muscle incision on the generation of guarding but normal heat and mechanical responses after skin only incision. On postoperative day 1, skin incision (53%) produced a similar prevalence of SA in dorsal horn neurons as the sham operated group

(36%), whereas skin plus deep tissue incision generated a greater prevalence of SA in dorsal horn neurons (78%); the rate of SA also tended to be greater after skin plus deep tissue incision (14 ± 3 imp/sec) versus the control group (6 ± 2) and skin incision group (9 ± 2 imp/sec). Seven days after skin plus deep tissue incision, when pain behaviors had resolved, the prevalence of SA (30%) and the amount of SA (6 ± 2) were similar as the sham group. Bupivacaine infiltration into the incision decreased SA in the skin plus deep tissue incision group to the same level as the sham operated rats on postoperative day 1 [23]. These data demonstrated incised deep tissue rather than skin had a central role in the genesis of guarding behavior and SA in nociceptors and nociceptive transmitting dorsal horn neurons. Nociceptor and dorsal horn SA was associated with guarding behavior after incision. Decreased heat withdrawal latency and decreased mechanical withdrawal threshold occurred with skin incision only.

4. Mechanisms of Pain Caused by a Surgical Incision

The patterns of pain behavior after surgical incisions in rodents indicate that peripheral and central sensitization occur. In neurophysiological experiments, activation and sensitization of peripheral nociceptors [6] and spinal dorsal horn neurons [9] were identified, and their specific mechanisms were investigated further.

4.1. Spinal Sensitization after Surgical Incision

It is very intriguing that spinal administration of many substances that are able to prevent central sensitization in other pain models failed to produce a significant effect after incision; the first studies in the plantar incision model indicated this using spinal N-methyl-D-aspartate (NMDA) receptor antagonists which basically failed to produce any effect [25]. These effects (or rather failure of effects) led to the assumption that an incision causes a different "form" of spinal sensitization compared to other pain entities. Additional pharmacological support for a unique spinal sensitization process after incision came from pharmacologic studies showing that non-NMDA/a-amino-3-hydroxy-5-methyl- 4-isoxazole propionate (AMPA) receptor antagonists are involved in the spinal transmission of pain behavior after incision [26]. This again differs from many other pain models and was somehow striking by firstly questioning the general "rule" of a NMDA receptor-dependent central sensitization process relevant for certain types of pain, e.g., after an incision and secondly "promoting" another rather new player in the game, namely the non-NMDA receptor group. The first issue was elaborated further by studies investigating the role of preemptive analgesia for PP, where NMDA receptors had earlier been identified as key molecules [27]. Spinal sensitization after the plantar incision is maintained (at least initially) by the afferent barrage of sensitized nociceptors and the non-NMDA/AMPA receptor group is maintaining this process which is responsible for nonevoked pain and hyperalgesia after incision [28]. More recent studies further elucidated mechanisms of AMPA-receptor mediated pain and hyperalgesia after incision and found that phosphorylation of the AMPA receptor GluR1 subunit at Serine-831 via phospho kinase C gamma (PKCg), but not other conventional PKC's isoforms (PKCa, βI and βII), leads to an increased trafficking of Ca^{2+} permeable AMPA receptors in the neuronal plasma membrane and might play a role for incisional pain. Interestingly, AMPA receptor phosphorylation was enhanced under (social defeat) stress after incision [29]; at the same time, incision-induced punctate mechanical hyperalgesia was prolonged. Besides phosphorylation of AMPA receptors, one subunit, GluR1, but not GluR2, is upregulated in the spinal cord ipsilateral to an incision. The regulation of the surface delivery of this spinal AMPA receptor subunit is caused by stargazin (member of the AMPA receptor regulatory protein family), and selective down-regulation of stargazin was able to reduce synaptic targeting of GluR1 subunit and nonevoked pain behavior and mechanical hyperalgesia caused by plantar incision. These spinal AMPA receptor subunits and the mechanisms regulating them after incision are therefore useful targets for drugs to treat pain after surgery in the future. However, spinal NMDA-receptor blockade might still have some indications. For example, remifentanil-induced enhanced mechanical hyperalgesia after incision in rats is regulated via phosphorylation of spinal NR2B at Tyr1472 which was prevented by ketamine.

This has clinical implications as discussed below. Studies showing different effects of spinal substances on different pain modalities are very interesting. Two examples are an effect on mechanical hyperalgesia, but not on nonevoked guarding pain and vice versa; and the activation of spinal aminobutyric acid (GABA)-receptors, especially GABAA and GABAB, attenuated the generation of mechanical/heat hyperalgesia but not nonevoked pain after plantar incision. Similarly, the selective inhibition of spinal pERK1/2 before incision exclusively altered mechanical hyperalgesia after incision but not nonevoked pain [30]. A comparable differentiation has been shown by Reichl et al. [31]; the inhibition of glutamate transporter (GluT) upregulation via mitogen-activated protein kinase p38 enhanced acute nonevoked pain after plantar incision, but did not alter mechanical or heat hyperalgesia. Interestingly, the effect of GluT inhibition extended the acute phase and lasted for approximately 2 weeks after incision. Thus, development of prolonged pain after surgery may be a result of impaired GLuT upregulation via p38 indicating a role spinal GluT in the prevention of chronic pain after incision. In the same way, prolonged pain behavior after the plantar incision was reported by inhibition of spinal cannabinoid receptors (CB1 and CB2) and dysregulation of mitogen-activated protein kinase phosphatase-3 [32]. Mitogenactivated protein kinase phosphatase-3 knockout mice showed a persistent mechanical hyperalgesia up to 21 days after surgical incision; this correlated with persistent phosphorylation of spinal p38 and extracellular signal-regulated kinases (ERKs)-1/2 in neurons and microglia on postoperative day 12. Together, these studies indicate the relevance of assessing the effect of various compounds after plantar incision in different pain behavior assays (nonevoked pain behavior, mechanical hyperalgesia), in particular to determine potential clinical relevance (resting pain vs movement evoked pain) after surgery

[33]. Secondly, these studies identify factors relevant for prolongation of incisional pain; this may translate to mechanisms relevant for the development of chronic pain after surgery, another important clinical issue [34].

Many other studies were undertaken to investigate pharmacological options to influence pain and hyperalgesia after incision by spinal modulation. For example, subcutaneous co-administration of morphine and gabapentin generates a dose-dependent antihyperalgesic synergistic effect [35]. Similarly, intrathecal administration of gabapentin together with diclofenac, in doses not affecting nociception, reduced secondary hyperalgesia after incision. Thus, diclofenac augments the antihyperalgesic effects of gabapentin through spinal action [36]. These findings highlight that certain combinations of medicines might offer benefits in the treatment of postsurgical pain and need to be assessed in future clinical studies.

4.2. Peripheral Sensitization after Incision

After plantar incision, peripheral C and Aδ fibers are sensitized contributing to nonevoked pain and heat and mechanical hyperalgesia in the early days after incision [37]. Some of the underlying mechanisms were investigated within the last 10 years. Combined behavioral and neurophysiological experiments revealed that muscle nociceptors play a central role in the genesis of nonevoked guarding behavior after incision; the mechanism seems to be the spontaneous activity of C fibers sensitized after incision [23, 24]. In contrast, a skin incision without a muscle tissue injury seems to be responsible for inducing mechanical hyperalgesia after incision; muscle injury seems to be not required [23, 24]. A series of studies revealed mechanisms inherent in (muscle) fiber sensitization after incision. They basically found a decrease in pH (pH; 6.8) and an increase in lactate concentration (6 mM) that correlated well with a peak in pain behaviors at 1 to 2 days after incision [38]. Similarly, a decrease of oxygen tension in both skeletal muscle and skin was detected immediately after incision for several days [39]; together with an increased lactate and decrease pH (see above), these ischemiclike conditions in the incisional wound are likely to contribute to peripheral sensitization (e.g., muscle C-fibers) and pain behavior (e.g., nonevoked pain) after incision. Furthermore, a response of muscle C-fibers to antagonists to acid-sensing ion channels (ASICs) in cultured dorsal root ganglion (DRG) neurons points towards the role of tissue acidity in nonevoked pain behavior after incision [40]. Interestingly, the ASIC3 channel is upregulated early after incision in muscle tissue innervating DRG neurons and seems to be important for nonevoked incisional pain, weight-bearing, and also partially for heat hyperalgesia. The role of ASIC3 for heat hyperalgesia is being controversially discussed in the literature with regard to different pain models. Whereas in vivo knockdown or specific inhibition via toxin APETx2a leads to complete remission of heat hyperalgesia after Complete Freund's Adjuvant (CFA) injection, mechanical but not heat hyperalgesia after carrageenan injection into the muscle seems to be ASIC3 mediated. Together, the role of ASIC (e.g., ASIC3) channel blocker for pain in general and specifically for incisional pain needs further investigation.

The role of specific peripheral mechanisms contributing to hyperalgesia after the incision has been investigated as well. There are 2 important aspects, which will be highlighted here: Firstly there are different nociceptors that seem to be responsible

for heat vs mechanical hyperalgesia after incision. Secondly, the molecular mechanisms of the fiber sensitization process responsible for mechanical and heat hyperalgesia after incision differ in many ways to other pain entities. Hints for the first aspect came from early studies using pretreatment of the incision site with a low dose of capsaicin (transient receptor potential vanilloid 1 receptor agonist); this reduced the heat hyperalgesia (and nonevoked pain) but not mechanical hyperalgesia after incision [21]. Consistent with other pain models, there is an upregulation of peripheral (and spinal) transient receptor potential vanilloid 1, which contributes to the development of heat (but not mechanical) hyperalgesia after incision [41]. There are many other examples differentiating mechanical and heat hyperalgesia after incision. One example for the second aspect, a differential sensitization process relevant for hyperalgesia after incision compared to inflammation or neuropathic pain, is the important role of calcitonin gene-related peptide in inflammation-related pain (CFA), which is not involved in spontaneous pain or mechanical and heat hyperalgesia after incision in mice. Further confirmation for an unique peripheral sensitization process after incision came from a study investigating 84 mRNAs from the neurotrophins and inflammatory cytokines families in skin, muscle, and DRG after plantar incision [42]. As demonstrated, most alterations in the mRNA expression are present in incised skin and muscle, less in the DRG. They occur within the first 48 hours after incision when the mechanical and heat hyperalgesia, as well as guarding pain, is most obvious. In particular, genes for wound healing, reinnervation, and the immune response are differently expressed in comparison to other pain models [42]. Only recently peripheral inflammatory cell responses were investigated after incision injury in animals. For instance, migration of neutrophilic granulocytes (NGs) into tissue traumatized by incision occurs shortly after surgery, reaching a maximum at 24 hours and declining rapidly to baseline within 3 days [43]. Neutrophilic granulocytess release many wellknown proinflammatory mediators and contain endogenous opioid peptides (met-enkephalin and b-endorphin) [44]. Sahbaie and colleagues demonstrated that the systemic depletion of NGs (with Gr-1 antibody) reduced the paw edema and the interleukin-1b (IL-1b) concentration, but increased significantly the heat hyperalgesia for 24 hours and did not alter the mechanical hyperalgesia after plantar incision in mice. This suggests a role of endogenous opioids (released by NGs) for incisional pain similar to that shown in inflammatory pain models [45]. However, another study used the same method to deplete NGs but showed attenuation of mechanical hyperalgesia after incision; they suggested the role of CXCL-1-CXCR1/2 recruitment of NGs after incision. Presumably, proinflammatory mediators from NGs (IL-1b and C5a) may play a role for hyperalgesia after incision [46]. Thus, as the local concentration of C5a after the incision is increased, this complement factor may provide a novel target for analgesic drug development. However, the exact role of NGs in postoperative pain is currently unclear because of the contradictory results of both NGdepletion studies [43]. The prevention of mast cell degranulation (mast cell membrane stabilization with Cromoglycate) or depletion of mast cell mediators (with Compound 48/80 prior to incision), thus inhibiting the effect of histamine, 5-HT, and tryptase (a serine protease localized exclusively in mast cells) reduce the mechanical hyperalgesia and nonevoked pain in mice. Similar effects are observed by administration of tryptase-binding receptor antagonist (protease-activated receptor 2, PAR2) [47]. These results suggest a role of mast cells contributing to hypersensitization after incision. However, it should be noted that the mast cell degranulation alone seems insufficient to promote pain (e.g., allergies, some drug administration).

4.3. Neuroplastic Changes in the Brain after Incision

Our understanding of the processing of pain in the human brain has improved significantly [48]; however, activity and neuroplasticity in the pain matrix after incision contributing to pain-related behavior remains poorly understood. A recent study in animals indicates directly how the brain reacts to an incision compared to inflammation by using functional magnetic resonance imaging to assess oxygenation levels of the blood as an indirect measure of neural activity and functional magnetic resonance spectroscopy [49]. Mechanical stimulation of the incised hind paw showed blood oxygen level dependent (BOLD) signals, which differed significantly in quantity and quality to BOLD signals related to mechanical stimulation of the hind paw after CFA inflammation. Similarly, BOLD signals after electrical stimulation in both animal models differed to mechanical stimulation. However, GABA levels (measured with functional magnetic resonance spectroscopy) increased in both pain models within the thalamus, during rest and during mechanical stimulation. Thus, the thalamus might play a central role for hyperalgesia regardless of the pain entity and GABA neurotransmission might be involved. Further imaging studies investigated central neuroplastic changes relevant for the development of more chronic pain after incision. Human functional magnetic resonance imaging studies confirmed the role the thalamus [50] and indicated a lack of descending inhibition in enhanced pain responses of patients with chronic pain after incision [51]. By using the positron emission tomography-method, Romero et al. [52] demonstrated long-lasting changes in glucose metabolism in central painrelated areas and opioid-related pathways up to 21 days after incision. The metabolic changes in the pain matrix were positively correlated with hypersensitivity caused by naloxone injection in rats which received remifentanil anesthesia earlier. This suggests long-lasting neuroplastic adaptations in central opioid circuits possibly contributing to chronic pain after incision. Systemic administration of gabapentin, or inhibition of ERK within the anterior cingulate cortex (ACC) early after surgery, but not systemic morphine, reduced incision-induced anxiety [53]. Interestingly, ERK-inhibition reduced anxiety-like behavior and mechanical hyperalgesia early after surgery (1 hour), but (different to inflammatory and neuropathic pain) in the later phase (6 hour), it exclusively reduced anxiety. A recent study showed that presurgical or postsurgical exposure to stress factors like immobilization and force swimming test does not change the basal pain perception to different stimuli, such as mechanical, hot and cold, but prolongs the duration of incision-induced hyperalgesia after incision [54]. By blocking spinal glucocorticoid receptors or removing the adrenal glands, stress-induced prolongation of incision-induced hyperalgesia was abrogated. These results indicate a direct connection between the activation of the hypothalamic-pituitary-adrenal axis through presurgery and postsurgery stress and duration of incision-induced hypersensitivities. Maternal adversity in the form of perinatal stress and depression may also activate the hypothalamic-pituitary-adrenal system and increased incisional pain in adult rats [55]. Thus, acute stress might be—similar to other psychological factors—relevant for the transformation of acute into chronic pain after surgery.

4.4. Epigenetic Modulation after Incision

In recent years, a growing body of publications has examined the potential of the epigenetic modulation, such as DNA methylation, histone acetylation and noncoding RNA, for chronic pain conditions. Some epigenetic results are now available for acute postoperative incisional pain in animals. An incision seems to induce changes in global DNA methylation, which leads to increased incision-induced hyperalgesia. Peripheral and spinal inhibition of a DNA methyltransferase via 5-Aza-2′-deoxycytidine led to attenuation of the mechanical and heat hyperalgesia and reduced hind paw swelling [56]. Furthermore, epigenetic modulation of spinal Bdnf2 (brain-derived neurotropic factor) and Pdyn2 (prodynorphin) genes via acetylated Histone H3K9 in mice under chronic opioid exposure seems to be involved in opioid tolerance after incision [57]. Notably, different histone deacetylase inhibitors, such as suberoylanilide hydroxamic acid or trichostatin A, attenuated heat hyperalgesia or mechanical hyperalgesia in an inflammatory (CFA) and in a neuropathic pain model, but exacerbated mechanical hyperalgesia after incision in mice. Taken together, these first epigenetic results suggest that peripheral and spinal epigenetic modulation are involved in increased postoperative nociceptive sensitization. The additional influence of epigenetic regulation by drugs (e.g., opioids) or environmental input could induce long-lasting changes in the pain system, one possible cause for a transformation from acute to chronic conditions.

REFERENCES

[1] Brennan TJ, Zahn PK, Pogatzki-Zahn EM. Mechanisms of incisional pain. *Anesthesiol Clin North America.* 2005;23(1):1-20.

[2] Rice AS, Cimino-Brown D, Eisenach JC, Kontinen VK, Lacroix-Fralish ML, Machin I, et al. Animal models and the prediction of efficacy in clinical trials of analgesic drugs: a critical appraisal and call for uniform reporting standards. *Pain.* 2008;139(2):243-7.

[3] Schmidt R, Schmelz M, Forster C, Ringkamp M, Torebjörk E, Handwerker H. Novel classes of responsive and unresponsive C nociceptors in human skin. *J Neurosci.* 1995;15(1 Pt 1):333-41.

[4] Liang YF, Haake B, Reeh PW. Sustained sensitization and recruitment of rat cutaneous nociceptors by bradykinin and a novel theory of its excitatory action. *J Physiol.* 2001;532(Pt 1):229-39.

[5] Brennan TJ, Vandermeulen EP, Gebhart GF. Characterization of a rat model of incisional pain. *Pain.* 1996;64(3):493-501.

[6] Pogatzki EM, Gebhart GF, Brennan TJ. Characterization of Adelta- and C-fibers innervating the plantar rat hindpaw one day after an incision. *J Neurophysiol.* 2002;87(2):721-31.

[7] Xu J, Richebe P, Brennan TJ. Separate groups of dorsal horn neurons transmit spontaneous activity and mechanosensitivity one day after plantar incision. *Eur J Pain.* 2009;13(8):820-8.

[8] Kawamata M, Watanabe H, Nishikawa K, Takahashi T, Kozuka Y, Kawamata T, et al. Different mechanisms of development and maintenance of experimental incision-induced hyperalgesia in human skin. *Anesthesiology.* 2002;97(3):550-9.

[9] Zahn PK, Brennan TJ. Primary and secondary hyperalgesia in a rat model for human postoperative pain. *Anesthesiology.* 1999; 90(3):863-72.

[10] Scherer M, Reichl SU, Augustin M, Pogatzki-Zahn EM, Zahn PK. The assessment of cold hyperalgesia after an incision. *Anesth Analg.* 2010;110(1):222-7.

[11] Pogatzki EM, Niemeier JS, Brennan TJ. Persistent secondary hyperalgesia after gastrocnemius incision in the rat. *Eur J Pain.* 2002;6(4):295-305.

[12] Kouya F, Iqbal Z, Charen D, Shah M, Banik RK. Evaluation of anxiety-like behaviour in a rat model of acute postoperative pain. *Eur J Anaesthesiol.* 2015;32(4):242-7.

[13] Li CQ, Zhang JW, Dai RP, Wang J, Luo XG, Zhou XF. Surgical incision induces anxiety-like behavior and amygdala sensitization: effects of morphine and gabapentin. *Pain Res Treat.* 2010; 2010:705874.

[14] Pogatzki EM, Raja SN. A mouse model of incisional pain. *Anesthesiology.* 2003;99(4):1023-7.

[15] Castel D, Willentz E, Doron O, Brenner O, Meilin S. Characterization of a porcine model of post-operative pain. *Eur J Pain.* 2014;18(4):496-505.

[16] Clarke H, Bonin RP, Orser BA, Englesakis M, Wijeysundera DN, Katz J. The prevention of chronic postsurgical pain using gabapentin and pregabalin: a combined systematic review and meta-analysis. *Anesth Analg.* 2012;115(2):428-42.

[17] Xu B, Guan XH, Yu JX, Lv J, Zhang HX, Fu QC, et al. Activation of spinal phosphatidylinositol 3-kinase/protein kinase B mediates pain behavior induced by plantar incision in mice. *Exp Neurol.* 2014;255:71-82.

[18] Ohri R, Wang JC, Blaskovich PD, Pham LN, Costa DS, Nichols GA, et al. Inhibition by local bupivacaine-releasing microspheres of acute postoperative pain from hairy skin incision. *Anesth Analg.* 2013; 117(3):717-30.

[19] Bessou P, Perl ER. Response of cutaneous sensory units with unmyelinated fibers to noxious stimuli. *J Neurophysiol.* 1969; 32(6):1025-43.

[20] Burgess PR, Perl ER. Myelinated afferent fibres responding specifically to noxious stimulation of the skin. *J Physiol.* 1967; 190(3):541-62.

[21] Hämäläinen MM, Gebhart GF, Brennan TJ. Acute effect of an incision on mechanosensitive afferents in the plantar rat hindpaw. *J Neurophysiol.* 2002;87(2):712-20.

[22] Pogatzki EM, Vandermeulen EP, Brennan TJ. Effect of plantar local anesthetic injection on dorsal horn neuron activity and pain behaviors caused by incision. *Pain.* 2002;97(1-2):151-61.

[23] Xu J, Brennan TJ. Comparison of skin incision vs. skin plus deep tissue incision on ongoing pain and spontaneous activity in dorsal horn neurons. *Pain.* 2009;144(3):329-39.

[24] Xu J, Brennan TJ. Guarding pain and spontaneous activity of nociceptors after skin versus skin plus deep tissue incision. *Anesthesiology.* 2010;112(1):153-64.

[25] Flatters SJ. Effect of analgesic standards on persistent postoperative pain evoked by skin/muscle incision and retraction (SMIR). *Neurosci Lett.* 2010;477(1):43-7.

[26] Zahn PK, Brennan TJ. Lack of effect of intrathecally administered N-methyl-D-aspartate receptor antagonists in a rat model for postoperative pain. *Anesthesiology.* 1998;88(1):143-56.

[27] Pogatzki-Zahn EM, Zahn PK. From preemptive to preventive analgesia. *Curr Opin Anaesthesiol.* 2006;19(5):551-5.

[28] Zahn PK, Pogatzki-Zahn EM, Brennan TJ. Spinal administration of MK-801 and NBQX demonstrates NMDA-independent dorsal horn sensitization in incisional pain. *Pain.* 2005;114(3):499-510.

[29] Li C, Yang Y, Liu S, Fang H, Zhang Y, Furmanski O, et al. Stress induces pain transition by potentiation of AMPA receptor phosphorylation. *J Neurosci.* 2014;34(41):13737-46.

[30] van den Heuvel I, Reichl S, Segelcke D, Zahn PK, Pogatzki-Zahn EM. Selective prevention of mechanical hyperalgesia after incision by spinal ERK1/2 inhibition. *Eur J Pain.* 2015;19(2):225-35.

[31] Reichl S, Segelcke D, Keller V, Jonas R, Boecker A, Wenk M, et al. Activation of glial glutamate transporter via MAPK p38 prevents enhanced and long-lasting non-evoked resting pain after surgical incision in rats. *Neuropharmacology.* 2016;105:607-17.

[32] Saha M, Skopelja S, Martinez E, Alvarez DL, Liponis BS, Romero-Sandoval EA. Spinal mitogen-activated protein kinase phosphatase-3 (MKP-3) is necessary for the normal resolution of mechanical allodynia in a mouse model of acute postoperative pain. *J Neurosci.* 2013;33(43):17182-7.

[33] Srikandarajah S, Gilron I. Systematic review of movement-evoked pain versus pain at rest in postsurgical clinical trials and meta-analyses: a fundamental distinction requiring standardized measurement. *Pain.* 2011;152(8):1734-9.

[34] Kehlet H, Jensen TS, Woolf CJ. Persistent postsurgical pain: risk factors and prevention. *Lancet.* 2006;367(9522):1618-25.

[35] Papathanasiou T, Juul RV, Heegaard AM, Kreilgaard M, Lund TM. Co-administration of morphine and gabapentin leads to dose

dependent synergistic effects in a rat model of postoperative pain. *Eur J Pharm Sci.* 2016;82:97-105.

[36] Narai Y, Imamachi N, Saito Y. Gabapentin augments the antihyperalgesic effects of diclofenac sodium through spinal action in a rat postoperative pain model. *Anesth Analg.* 2012;115(1):189-93.

[37] Banik RK, Brennan TJ. Sensitization of primary afferents to mechanical and heat stimuli after incision in a novel in vitro mouse glabrous skin-nerve preparation. *Pain.* 2008;138(2):380-91.

[38] Woo YC, Park SS, Subieta AR, Brennan TJ. Changes in tissue pH and temperature after incision indicate acidosis may contribute to postoperative pain. *Anesthesiology.* 2004;101(2):468-75.

[39] Kang S, Lee D, Theusch BE, Arpey CJ, Brennan TJ. Wound hypoxia in deep tissue after incision in rats. *Wound Repair Regen.* 2013;21(5):730-9.

[40] Kido K, Gautam M, Benson CJ, Gu H, Brennan TJ. Effect of deep tissue incision on pH responses of afferent fibers and dorsal root ganglia innervating muscle. *Anesthesiology.* 2013;119(5):1186-97.

[41] Pogatzki-Zahn EM, Shimizu I, Caterina M, Raja SN. Heat hyperalgesia after incision requires TRPV1 and is distinct from pure inflammatory pain. *Pain.* 2005;115(3):296-307.

[42] Spofford CM, Brennan TJ. Gene expression in skin, muscle, and dorsal root ganglion after plantar incision in the rat. *Anesthesiology.* 2012;117(1):161-72.

[43] Carreira EU, Carregaro V, Teixeira MM, Moriconi A, Aramini A, Verri WA, et al. Neutrophils recruited by CXCR1/2 signalling mediate post-incisional pain. *Eur J Pain.* 2013;17(5):654-63.

[44] Rittner HL, Machelska H, Stein C. Leukocytes in the regulation of pain and analgesia. *J Leukoc Biol.* 2005;78(6):1215-22.

[45] Rittner HL, Labuz D, Schaefer M, Mousa SA, Schulz S, Schäfer M, et al. Pain control by CXCR2 ligands through Ca2+-regulated release of opioid peptides from polymorphonuclear cells. *FASEB J.* 2006;20(14):2627-9.

[46] Jang JH, Liang D, Kido K, Sun Y, Clark DJ, Brennan TJ. Increased local concentration of complement C5a contributes to incisional pain in mice. *J Neuroinflammation.* 2011;8:80.

[47] Oliveira SM, Silva CR, Ferreira J. Critical role of protease-activated receptor 2 activation by mast cell tryptase in the development of postoperative pain. *Anesthesiology.* 2013;118(3):679-90.

[48] Maihöfner C, Seifert F, Decol R. Activation of central sympathetic networks during innocuous and noxious somatosensory stimulation. *Neuroimage.* 2011;55(1):216-24.

[49] Amirmohseni S, Segelcke D, Reichl S, Wachsmuth L, Görlich D, Faber C, et al. Characterization of incisional and inflammatory pain in rats using functional tools of MRI. *Neuroimage.* 2016;127:110-22.

[50] Pogatzki-Zahn EM, Wagner C, Meinhardt-Renner A, Burgmer M, Beste C, Zahn PK, et al. Coding of incisional pain in the brain: a functional magnetic resonance imaging study in human volunteers. *Anesthesiology.* 2010;112(2):406-17.

[51] Burgmer M, Pfleiderer B, Maihöfner C, Gaubitz M, Wessolleck E, Heuft G, et al. Cerebral mechanisms of experimental hyperalgesia in fibromyalgia. *Eur J Pain.* 2012;16(5):636-47.

[52] Romero A, Rojas S, Cabañero D, Gispert JD, Herance JR, Campillo A, et al. A ^{18} F-fluorodeoxyglucose MicroPET imaging study to assess changes in brain glucose metabolism in a rat model of surgery-induced latent pain sensitization. *Anesthesiology.* 2011; 115(5):1072-83.

[53] Dai RP, Li CQ, Zhang JW, Li F, Shi XD, Zhang JY, et al. Biphasic activation of extracellular signal-regulated kinase in anterior cingulate cortex distinctly regulates the development of pain-related anxiety and mechanical hypersensitivity in rats after incision. *Anesthesiology.* 2011;115(3):604-13.

[54] Cao J, Wang PK, Tiwari V, Liang L, Lutz BM, Shieh KR, et al. Short-term pre- and post-operative stress prolongs incision-induced pain hypersensitivity without changing basal pain perception. *Mol Pain.* 2015;11:73.

evolve into chronic pain syndrome, reduced cardiac output, dizziness, somnolence and short-duration central muscle stiffness. Opioid induced ventilatory impairment is well known by anesthesiologists and is easily treated in the post-anesthesia care unit, but this complication is still problematic postoperatively, especially in the bariatric surgery population. Another side effect is pharyngeal muscle weakness, contributing to obstructive breathing patterns in every patient. This side effect should certainly be avoided in obese patients and patients with obstructive sleep apnea (OSA), given the potential for aggravation and further breathing obstruction. Accordingly recommendations for anesthesiologists are to avoid or minimize the perioperative use of opioids in these patients.

If no opioids are used during surgery, fewer opioids are needed to achieve a pain-free recovery, as addiction has not yet destroyed the mu receptor system. Opioid induced hyperalgesia and chronic pain syndromes are more frequent when high-dose opioids are used perioperatively [1].

Thoracic Epidural Analgesia (TEA)

Initiation of neuroaxial blockade before surgery and its maintenance throughout surgery decreases the need for anesthetic agents, opioids and muscle relaxants. Compared with parenteral opioids, epidural blockade has shown to provide better postoperative static and dynamic analgesia for the first 72 h, to accelerate the recovery of gastrointestinal function, to reduce insulin resistance and impact positively on cardiovascular and respiratory complications.

However, it also has side effects like: hypotension, urinary retention, pruritus and motor blockade. Although detrusor function can be impaired in patients receiving this technique, it has been shown that early removal of a urinary catheter (on postoperative day 1) does not increase the risk of bladder recatheterization and urinary infection.

The same benefits have not been observed after laparoscopic procedures, especially in a context of an ERAS program. However, thoracic epidural analgesia might still be valuable in patients at risk of respiratory complications, or in those with high probability of conversion to laparotomy.

Continuous Wound Infusion

Continuous wound infusion of local anesthetic after open abdominal surgery has been shown to improve postoperative analgesia and reduce opioid consumption. Regarding laparoscopic abdominal surgery, it has been demonstrated that pain intensity was similar among patients receiving epidural and wound infusion of local anesthetic.

Despite these promising results, there are several aspects related to this techniques which need to be clarified. It remains to be established if the analgesic effect observed in these trials is mainly driven by the bolus of local anesthetic given at the end of surgery of by the infusion of local anesthetic during the postoperative period.

TAP Block

Significant reduction of pain intensity and opioid consumption after ultrasound-guided single-shot TAP block has been observed but it is limited to the first 24 hours after surgery. TAP blocks can also be performed by surgeons from the peritoneal cavity before closing the abdominal wall, or laparoscopic guided. Only few studies have reported a reduction of some of the opioid side effects, but these results have not been reproduced consistently.

Optimal timing, choice of local anesthetic, dosing and volumes remain unknown. However, it seems that a minimal volume of 15 ml is required to achieve satisfactory analgesia with single-shot TAP block. Ropivacaine 0.2% (8–10 ml/h) can be infused for 48–72 h through a multihole catheter.

Intraperitoneal Local Anesthesia

It has been shown to improve postoperative analgesia, reduce shoulder pain and opioid consumption after laparoscopic gastric surgery.

Opioids

The primary objective should be to minimize or avoid the use of opioids wherever possible. Under general anesthesia, patients are unconscious and do not perceive pain. Although there is no pain perception, surgery induced activation of nociceptive reflex arcs has hemodynamic consequences. Using opioids to reduce the hemodynamic changes should be resisted as much as possible, as hyperalgesia can develop acutely and opioid-related side effects can occur at very low doses.

Control of blood pressure and heart rate at intubation and during surgery by beta-blockers, calcium channel blockers, or lidocaine should be encouraged rather than using opioids without a specific indication other than intraoperative tachycardia or hypertension [4].

Multimodal Analgesia

A multimodal analgesia regimen is based on routine use of NSAID's and paracetamol (PO o intravenously). It should be adopted if not contraindicated in patients undergoing open or laparoscopic bariatric surgery with the aim to reduce opioid consumption and their dose-dependent side effects that impair recovery.

Acetaminophen (paracetamol) has shown to improve postoperative analgesia, have an opioid-sparing effect, but not to reduce opioids side effects.

Concerns have been raised about the cardiovascular risk and delayed bone healing associated with the use of NSAID's and COX-2 inhibitors.

The evidence is inconclusive and does not support the avoidance of short perioperative treatment in patients with low cardiovascular risk.

High-dose of systemic steroids have also shown promising results, when used carefully in patients undergoing gastrointestinal surgery. Perioperative intravenous ketamine and gabapentinoids have also shown opioid sparing properties. However, the risk of side effects such as dizziness and sedation should be considered.

Gabapentin or pregabalin should be considered as part of a multimodal analgesia protocol. Both medications are associated with reduced opioid requirements and appear effective when administered as a preoperative dose. It is difficult to determine optimal doses, because higher doses might be more effective, but they might also be associated with more sedation. They are only available in oral form, potentially limiting their use in the immediate postoperative period. Dose reductions are recommended in patients with impaired renal function.

Intravenous ketamine has been evaluated as a part of multimodal analgesia. It has been found in several studies that ketamine IV infusions were associated with decreased postoperative pain medications use compared with placebo, and with a decreased risk of persistent postsurgical pain. If administered perioperatively, ketamine is associated with increased risk of hallucinations and nightmares.

Glucocorticoid steroids may have analgesic properties possibly related to anti-inflammatory properties and should be considered as part of a multimodal perioperative pain protocol. The concern for significant hyperglycemia (>180 mg/dL) in bariatric patients has not been confirmed [3].

Dexmedetomidine is a highly selective α2-agonist. It is approximately 8 times more specific to α2 adrenergic receptors than clonidine and its elimination half-life is much shorter. This medication should be administered cautiously as several cardiovascular effects may occur. For example, dexmedetomidine should be given over at least 10 minutes, as hypertensive episodes may otherwise be provoked. Nonetheless, a generally hypotensive effect of dexmedetomidine (as well as clonidine) may be observed later as well. In addition, bradycardia may commonly occur, and even cases of asystole have been reported. Importantly, the use of dexmedetomidine is contraindicated in patients with higher degree AV-blocks. While there are certainly many benefits associated with the use of dexmedetomidine in the perioperative setting, caution is required [6].

Intravenous Lidocaine

In view of its antinociceptive and anti-inflammatory properties, systemic administration of lidocaine as adjuvant to systemic opioids has been shown to improve postoperative analgesia, reduce opioid consumption and speed surgical recovery.

Side effects are directly related to serum levels, and are more pronounced in patients with liver dysfunction, pulmonary diseases when the predominant problem is carbon dioxide retention, and congestive heart failure [4].

Intraoperative Clinical Management

Gabapentin 150–300 mg can be given as premedication orally and continued the next day postoperatively, when the patient can take oral medication. Dexmedetomidine loading dose of 0.25 µg/kg is given 15 minutes before induction. The dose is further increased to 0.5 or 1 µg/kg and continued with 0.5–1 µg/kg/h, if the procedure takes longer than two hours. Rapid awakening requires the use of the lowest possible dexmedetomidine dose (<0.5 µg/kg), frequently without maintenance doses.

Clonidine has a much longer half-life and is therefore less suitable for short procedures.

Lidocaine 1.5 mg/kg and magnesium 40 mg/kg given at induction and by infusion (lidocaine or procaine 1–3 mg/kg/h and magnesium 5–15 mg/kg/h) further improve the multimodal approach.

Ketorolac (0.5 mg/kg) or diclofenac (150mg) and dexamethasone (10 mg) should be administered before surgery to reduce inflammation. The use of propofol combined with a sympathetic block is possible but requires high propofol doses, while inhalational anesthetics can be given below one minimum alveolar concentration value.

Most of these doses are calculated for lean body weight or ideal body weight +20%, which is easier to calculate instead of total body weight [1].

Postoperative Clinical Management

Epidural blockade should be tested before surgery or in the immediate postoperative period to avoid non-functioning epidurals and unnecessary opioid administration. The addition of opioids to local anesthetic has shown to improve postoperative analgesia. Although epidural solution containing morphine increases the risk of urinary retention.

However, the use of low dose of local anesthetics (bupivacaine 0.1 mg/ml) and lipophilic opioids (e.g., fentanyl) seem to provide optimal analgesia with minimal side effects. Epidural morphine in adjunct to local anesthetic can be preferred to lipophilic opioids to increase segmental analgesia spread and could be recommended for long midline incisions. Epidural infusions can be continued for 48-72, gradually reducing infusion rates and until the recovery of gastrointestinal function.

Adding adrenaline (1.5–2.0 lg/ml) to epidural mixture of local anesthetic and fentanyl improves postoperative analgesia, especially during mobilization and coughing, and reduces pruritus and nausea.

Hypotension induced by epidural blockade should be treated with vasopressors as first choice provided the patient is not hypovolaemic. Orthostatic hypotension associated with postoperative epidural analgesia does not impair the ability to ambulate [2].

When waking the patient up, give a loading dose of paracetamol and continue with paracetamol 1gr every 6 hours for several days, if needed. Add a non-steroidal anti-inflammatory drug (NSAID) such as diclofenac

(75 mg every 12 hours) for up to the first two days. Continue with oral gabapentine (150-300 mg / day) when possible.

Continue the sympathetic block by loading up with an extra dose of clonidine (75-150 μg), lidocaine 1 mg/Kg, and ketamine 25 mg at the end of anesthesia if not already done.

It is better to keep giving these in a continuous infusion bag or pump over the next 10-24 hours. Medication choices for infusion include clonidine (0,1 μg/Kg/h) or dexmedetomidine (0,1 μg/Kg/h), ketamine (0,05 mg/Kg/h) and magnesium (5 mg/Kg/h).

Dexmedetomidine and procaine are shorter acting and therefore preferable. A continuous infusion of dexmedetomidine, magnesium, ketamine or lidocaine might require follow-up on a high dependency care unit.

The exact duration of the lidocaine infusion providing optimal analgesia and facilitating also recovery remains unknown. Systemic toxicity is rare, but continuous cardiovascular monitoring is required.

Be aware that although most of these drugs are given postoperatively below sedation levels, dose reduction may be required if residual sedation persists postoperatively in older and frail patients [1].

Opioid Analgesia

Although one of the main analgesic goals for the bariatric surgery today is minimization of opioid use, one must recognize that opioids are still an important analgesic option. However, their role is less central when compared to traditional care where opioids where the main analgesic options for postoperative pain management.

For opioid-naïve patients who are not yet tolerating oral intake, patients ideally would have one of the main local anesthetic based options and multimodal analgesia before utilizing short-acting IV opioids for rescue analgesia. After these, opioid-naïve patients are tolerating oral intake, then short-acting oral opioids can be added for breakthrough pain after a scheduled regimen of nonopioid analgesics such as gabapentin, acetaminophen, NSAIDs, and other multimodal analgesic agents.

Thus, although some chronic pain patients will benefit from a PCA, the assumption that IV opioids via PCA should be a standard part of postoperative recovery is not necessarily valid in this case, and should be reconsidered [5].

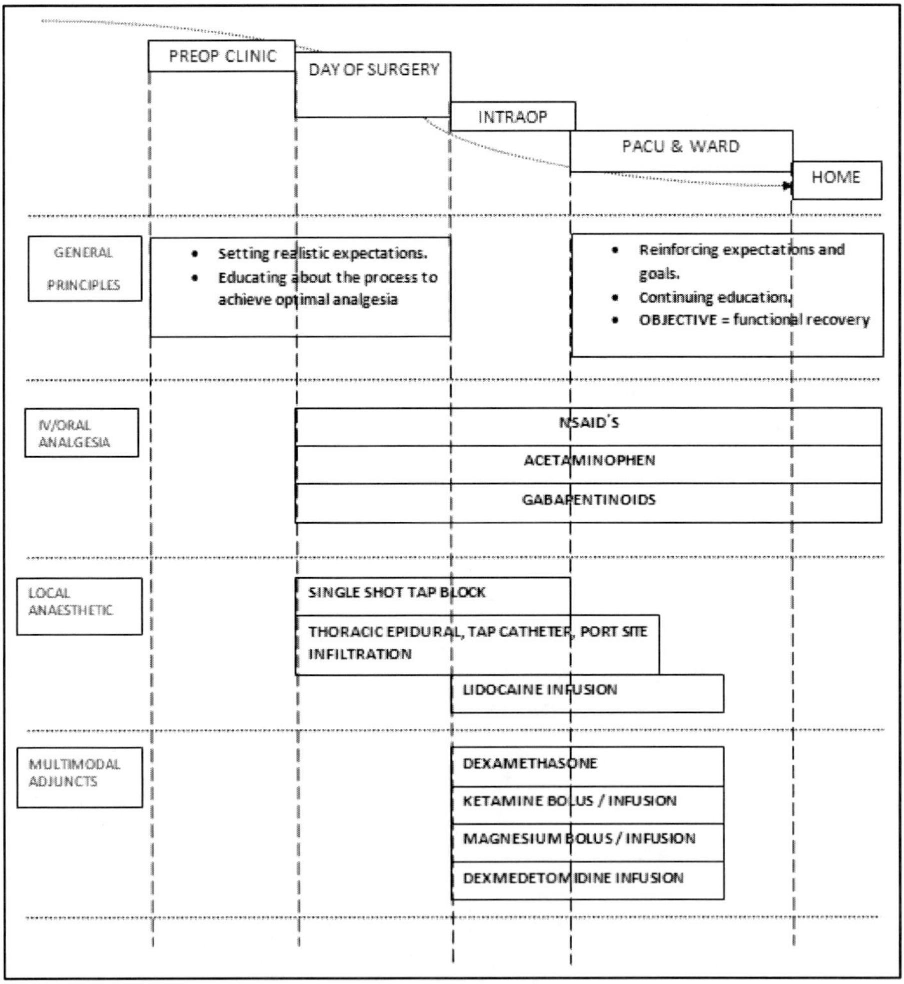

Figure 1. Analgesia scheme for bariatric surgery patients.

KEY POINTS

1. Thoracic epidural analgesia (T6-T11) still remains the gold standard for postoperative pain control in patients undergoing open bariatric surgery.
2. Patients scheduled for gastric bypass surgery or sleeve gastrectomy are often enrolled in an opioid free regimen. This protocols combine several non-opioid analgesic treatments in order to eliminate, or at least minimize opioid dosing. In the case of laparoscopic bariatric surgery this works remarkably well.
3. These regimens include drugs that can stabilize the sympathetic nervous system, including alpha-2 agonists (clonidine and dexmedetomidine), locoregional anesthetics given intravenously (lidocaine or procaine), magnesium, and gamma-aminobutyric acid modulators (gabapentin).
4. Regional techniques may also play an important role. A transversus abdominis plane block is an efferent block of the anterior abdominal wall that could reduce pain when employed in the context of multimodal analgesia.
5. Other components of the analgesic schemes for bariatric surgery are: ketamine, acetaminophen, NSAID's and glucocorticoids.
6. If an opioid must be used, it is recommended to use small doses of short-acting opioids such as alfentanil or fentanyl.

REFERENCES

[1] Mulier J. Opioid free general anesthesia: A paradigm shift? *Rev Esp Anestesiol Reanim*. 2017 Oct; 64(8):427-430.

[2] Feldheiser A, Aziz O2, Baldini G, Cox BP, Fearon KC, Feldman LS, Gan TJ, Kennedy RH, Ljungqvist O, Lobo DN, Miller T, Radtke FF, Ruiz Garces T, Schricker T, Scott MJ, Thacker JK, Ytrebø LM, Carli F. Enhanced Recovery After Surgery (ERAS) for gastrointestinal

surgery, part 2: consensus statement for anaesthesia practice. *Acta Anaesthesiol Scand.* 2016 Mar; 60(3):289-334.

[3] Chou R, Gordon DB, de Leon-Casasola OA, Rosenberg JM, Bickler S, Brennan T, Carter T, Cassidy CL, Chittenden EH, Degenhardt E, Griffith S, Manworren R, McCarberg B, Montgomery R, Murphy J, Perkal MF, Suresh S, Sluka K, Strassels S, Thirlby R, Viscusi E, Walco GA, Warner L, Weisman SJ, Wu CL. Management of Postoperative Pain: A Clinical Practice Guideline From the American Pain Society, the American Society of Regional Anesthesia and Pain Medicine, and the American Society of Anesthesiologists' Committee on Regional Anesthesia, Executive Committee, and Administrative Council. *J Pain.* 2016 Feb; 17(2):131-57.

[4] McEvoy MD, Scott MJ, Gordon DB, Grant SA, Thacker JKM, Wu CL, Gan TJ, Mythen MG, Shaw AD, Miller TE. Perioperative Quality Initiative (POQI) I Workgroup. American Society for Enhanced Recovery (ASER) and Perioperative Quality Initiative (POQI) joint consensus statement on optimal analgesia within an enhanced recovery pathway for colorectal surgery: part 1-from the preoperative period to PACU. *Perioper Med (Lond).* 2017 Apr 13; 6:8.

[5] Scott MJ, McEvoy MD, Gordon DB, Grant SA, Thacker JKM, Wu CL, Gan TJ, Mythen MG, Shaw AD, Miller TE. Perioperative Quality Initiative (POQI) I Workgroup. American Society for Enhanced Recovery (ASER) and Perioperative Quality Initiative (POQI) Joint Consensus Statement on Optimal Analgesia within an Enhanced Recovery Pathway for Colorectal Surgery: Part 2-From PACU to the Transition Home. *Perioper Med (Lond).* 2017 Apr 13; 6:7.

[6] Mauermann E, Ruppen W, Bandschapp O. Different protocols used today to achieve total opioid-free general anesthesia without loco-regional blocks, *Best Pract Res Clin Anaesthesiol.* 2017; doi: 10.1016/j.bpa.2017.11.003.

In: Management of Postoperative Pain … ISBN: 978-1-53614-284-6
Editor: Jaime Ruiz-Tovar

Chapter 3

MULTIMODAL ANALGESIA AND ADJUVANT ANALGESIC TREATMENT IN BARIATRIC SURGERY

Carmen Vallejo Lantero*[*], *MD* and *Esther García Villabona, MD
Anesthesiology Department. Hospital Universitario de La Princesa, Madrid, Spain

ABSTRACT

Increasing numbers of patients with morbid obesity are presenting for surgery and their acute pain management requires an evidence-based clinical update. The pathophysiology of obesity, typical co-morbidities and the high prevalence of obstructive sleep apnea make safe analgesic management difficult in these patients. Multimodal, evidence-based and procedure-specific analgesic regimens should be standard of care, with the aim to achieve optimal analgesia with minimal side effects. The perioperative use of non-opioid adjuvants appears to offer further improvements in patient's safety and outcomes.

[*] Corresponding Author Email: c.vallejo_26@hotmail.com.

Keywords: multimodal analgesia, adjuvant analgesics, pain management, bariatric surgery, obesity, postoperative pain, opioid-sparing

INTRODUCTION

With increasing awareness of both short- and long-term problems associated with liberal perioperative opioid administration, the need for routinely and clinically feasible alternatives is greater than ever. Opioids still represent the mainstay of any perioperative analgesic treatment plan. However, opioids can provoke severe side effects. Some of these side effects like postoperative nausea and vomiting (PONV) are obvious; others are not so manifest. Hyperalgesia and postoperative respiratory depression caused by opioids are of concern, yet often go unnoticed. Postoperative desaturation episodes are far more prevalent than generally appreciated, especially in patient groups with specific risk factors like morbid obesity (MO) or obstructive sleep apnea (OSA). Furthermore, undesirable side effects like constipation, urinary retention, and drowsiness may significantly impede an uneventful postoperative course [1].

In the obese patient, the goal of postoperative pain management is provision of comfort, early mobilization and improved respiratory function without causing inadequate sedation and respiratory compromise. The pathophysiology of obesity, typical co-morbidities and the high prevalence of OSA amongst obese patients make safe analgesic management difficult. In particular, pain control after bariatric surgery is a major challenge [2].

In times of ever more ERAS® (enhanced recovery after surgery) protocols emerging, the primary reliance on analgesic agents with such suboptimal side effect profile seems out-of-date. Although an opioid-free anesthesia and analgesia regimen long seemed elusive, newer truly multimodal protocols enable opioid-free (or at least opioid-sparing) anesthesia for certain types of operations. Multimodal, evidence-based and procedure-specific analgesic regimens should be standard of care, with the aim to achieve optimal analgesia with minimal side effects [3]. In patients with MO, these specific outcomes would also not be desirable, they are probably essential.

Though overall evidence is limited, multimodal analgesia with a step-wise, severity- based, opioid-sparing approach appears to improve acute pain management in morbid obesity. The perioperative use of non-opioid adjuvants appears to offer further improvements in patient's safety and outcomes [4].

Goals of Postoperative Analgesia in Morbid Obesity

Pain management of the obese patient in the perioperative setting is of great importance for not only the comfort, but also the outcome of patients. After bariatric surgery, pain is the most frequent postoperative problem, even if this surgery was performed laparoscopically. Adequate analgesia provides comfort for patients and this is an important treatment goal, but analgesia should also allow early mobilization, which, in turn, reduces the risk of deep vein thrombosis (DVT), pressure ulcers and respiratory complications including pneumonia [2].

The main risks for this patient group are perceived to be respiratory complications [5]. In MO, conventional opioid-based acute pain during intraoperative and post-operative pain management is associated with the risk of sedation, airway obstruction, and respiratory depression. Site of surgery (bariatric surgery) and co-existing OSA, which is very common in this population, are risk factors contributing to the increased incidence of pulmonary complications in obese patients [6]. Goals of postoperative analgesia should be the ability to comply with respiratory physiotherapy and early mobilization.

Multimodal Analgesia in Obese Patient

The concept of multimodal analgesia was introduced more than a decade ago as a technique to improve analgesia and reduce the incidence of opioid-related adverse events. Multimodal techniques for pain management include the administration of two or more drugs that act by different mechanisms for providing analgesia. These drugs may be administered via the same route or by different routes.

Multimodal analgesia involves the concurrent use of primarily non-opioid analgesics to take advantage of the additive, if not synergistic, effects that produce superior analgesia while decreasing opioid use and opioid-related side effects. Also, a key component of multimodal pain management is the utilization of regional analgesic techniques, including peripheral and field blocks and neuraxial blocks [7]. Recent data on the efficacy and safety of multimodal pain management strategies for weight loss surgery are consistent with this accepted approach of opioid-sparing postoperative analgesia in the general surgical patient population [8].

The ASA task force on acute pain management in 2012 recommended that multimodal pain analgesia should be included for the management of perioperative pain whenever possible [9]. It is widely accepted adjuvants such as ketamine, lidocaine and pregabalin, directed to avoid acute hyperalgesia, plays a major role in the treatment of acute pain in MO.

Acute Pain Management in Obese Patient

The role of multimodal analgesia and non-opioid adjuvant therapy has been shown to be beneficial in a variety of procedure-specific postoperative pain management protocols.

Acute pain management modalities can be divided into systemic analgesics and regional anesthesia techniques. The systemic analgesics have been further described as per the World Health Organization (WHO) Step Ladder approach- foundational, intermediate, opioid and adjuvant analgesics. This stepwise, severity based, opioid-sparing approach will be useful in all patients; more so in those with MO.

Systemic Medications

Acetaminophen and NSAIDs

Non opioid analgesics should be considered wherever possible.

- *Acetaminophen* is an important foundational World Health Organization (WHO) Step I whose mechanism of action is still not completely understood. It is highly selective and has an additive and not necessarily synergistic effect when combined with NSAIDs. It has been repeatedly shown to decrease opiod requirements in the perioperative setting and even contribute to shorter length of stay. The half-life of paracetamol does not change in obese patients, and plasma concentration measurements suggest that dosing according to the ideal weight is appropriate. IV acetaminophen is an attractive option in the perioperative period. It can be administered independent of enteral intake. *(Recommendation Grade B) [4].*
- *Ketorolac.* Cyclo-oxygenase inhibitors, as well non-selective NSAIDs such as selective coxibs, are the most widely used component of multimodal analgesia. The non-steroidal anti-inflammatory drugs are highly effective analgesics with the lowest numbers needed to treat (NNT) of all classes. Ketorolac administered regularly post-operatively can result in lower opioid consumption in patients with MO *(Recommendation Grade C)* [4]. The perioperative use of ketorolac alone or in combination with local anesthesia leads to significant improvement of postoperative pain control [2]. Similarly, an intraoperative infusion of ketorolac reduced pain scores and decreasing the incidence of postoperative nausea and vomiting (PONV).

Further studies of dose, safety and side effects specific to MO are needed.

Intermediate Analgesics: Tramadol and Tapentadol

Tramadol and Tapentadol are both intermediate-potency (WHO Step II) analgesics that may benefit surgical patients due to their multimodal mechanisms of action. Tramadol may be particularly useful when combined with acetaminophen *(Recommendation Grade B)* [4].

The use of tapentadol has not been yet reported specifically in this patient population. This is a newer molecule, related to tramadol but promisingly lacks the serotonergic effects of the latter, so reducing nausea, vomiting and interactions with anti-depressant medications.

Opioids Analgesics

Use of opioids for post-operative pain in patients with MO presents a challenge. Nevertheless, to achieve satisfactory pain control in obese patients after surgery, the employment of opioids is in some cases inevitable. Through the review of the literature base on the evidence available for the management of acute pain on MO, the current recommendations conclude that in case of use of opioid, PCA should be limited to patients with moderate to severe postoperative pain, probably when oral opioid therapy is not possible. Basal or continuous opioid infusions in patients with MO and particularly those with undiagnosed or untreated OSA should be avoided. Patients with suspected sleep disordered breathing must be observed with overnight monitoring of respiratory adequacy, during the entire time PCA is used *(Recommendation Grade C)* [4].

Adjuvants Analgesics

Gabanoids: Pregabalin/Gabapentina

Gabanoids, gabapentin and pregabalin, are anticonvulsants but are also called neuromodulators, as they reduce neuronal excitability by inhibiting the α-2-δ subunit of calcium-gated channels on presynaptic axons. Both of them plays a role as a component of multimodal analgesia in non obese patients. In MO patients, single preoperative adminstration of 150 mg pregabalin resulted in improved analgesia, opioid-sparing and reduced adverse effects such as nausea and vomiting [2]. Similarly, preoperative administration of 100 mg of gabapentin also produced significantly lower pain scores in recovery with less nausea-vomiting compared with placebo. However, pregabalin and gabapentin may be associated with increased sedation and postoperative respiratory depression.

There is no consensus for dose, frecuency or duration treatment. Their use in the perioperative period requires careful assessment of the risk-benefit in patients with MO and/or OSA *(Recommendation Grade C)* [4].

Nevertheless, although several single clinical trials report that gabanoids decrease the postoperative use of opioids, the Pfizer multi-centric phase III program failed to confirm these findings and to demonstrate any effectiveness in three different models. Nevertheless, the use of gabanoids for acute pain is extensive, even if it is not an approved indication. Recently, the non-approved use of gabanoids has been questioned [7].

NMDA Antagonist

With the discovery of the N-methyl-D-aspartate (NMDA) receptor and its links to nociceptive pain transmission and central sensitization, there has been renewed interest in utilizing noncompetitive NMDA receptor antagonists as potential antihyperalgesic agents.

Ketamine, magnesium, methadone, and dexamethasone all have NMDA-blocking ability, but ketamine has emerged as a frontrunner in the perioperative period [7].

- *Ketamine* has been a well known general anesthetic and analgesic drug. A review of available trials concluded that ketamine alone or added to morphine/hydromorphone showed mild improvement in postoperative analgesia while reducing opioid requirements along with reducing postoperative nausea and vomiting (PONV) [10].

An IV bolus before incision and then a continuous infusion is an effective option for postoperative pain control. If the infusion is administered over a prolonged period of time (48 hours) for more invasive and routinely painful procedures, patients can be at lower risk for developing persistent postoperative pain in the subsequent months. Low doses of ketamine (0,1-0,5 mg/kg) used in morbid obese lead to a significant reduced opioid consumption and reduced need for rescue analgesia importantly *(Recommendation Grade C)* [4]. Limiting factors for ketamine are co-existing severe arterial hypertension and cardiac failure, although the induction of hypertension by low-dose ketamine is unlikely.

- *Magnesium:* The magnesium ion was the first agent discovered to be an NMDA channel blocker. At very high doses, perioperative intravenous magnesium sulfate has been reported to reduce postoperative morphine consumption but not postoperative pain scores. However, as the magnesium ion crosses the blood–brain barrier poorly in humans, it is not clear whether the therapeutic effect is related to the NMDA antagonist effect studied in the central nervous system [11].

Alpha-2 Adrenergic Agonists

Alpha-2 adrenergic activation represents an intrinsic pain control network of the central nervous system. In bariatric surgery it was demonstrated that the use of alpha2-agonists leads to a reduction in postoperative opioid consumption, less respiratory depression, shorter PACU stay, less use of antiemetics, and a favourable cardiovascular stability.

- *Dexmedetomidine* is an α 2 receptor agonist with sedative and analgesic sparing properties. Various studies in MO population have shown safety of dexmedetomidine infusion perioperatively and the capacity to minimize narcotic requeriments, length of stay after laparoscopic bariatric procedures and the risk of developing PONV *(Recommendation Grade B)* [4,12].

- *Clonidine.* Due to the many side effects of systemic clonidine administration (hypotension, bradycardia, and sedation), the spinal route is preferred. When clonidine is used as a premedication, it has found to be more sedating and associated with bradycardia and hypotension. Clonidine has been used in a limited number of studies in patients with MO.

When comparing pain scores, quantity of analgesic consumption, PONV and patient satisfaction, a single study reported comparable benefits between clonidine and dexmedetomidine [4]. Up to date it remains unclear if there is a clinical difference between the two substances, of which dexmedetomidine possesses a much higher specificity of the alpha2-adrenoceptor. Optimal dosing strategies are lacking providing the best balance between perioperative analgesia, patient safety, and quick recovery. Nonetheless alpha2-agonist appear to be one of the most tempting tools in the anaesthesiologist's arsenal to reduce perioperative opioid consumption [11].

Lidocaine

Lidocaine has analgesic effect, anti-hyperalgesic and anti-inflammatory properties, which makes it use as a general anesthetic adjuvant. Lidocaine is capable of reducing nociception and/or cardiovascular responses to the surgical stress, and postoperative pain and/or analgesic requirements. If the exact mechanism of action remains not fully explained; bolus then continuous lidocaine infusion has clear analgesic benefits. Lidocaine is one of major drug for opioid reduced anesthesia (ORA) or opioid free anesthesia (OFA) procedures. It clearly improves the postoperative outcomes with increased patient satisfaction. Such procedure takes place wisely in the ERAS protocols [13]. With recommended protocols, safety will be as great as his efficacy. Very little information is available in patients with morbid obesity indicating a significant decrease in opioid consumption in PACU and at 24 hours post analgesia regimen *(Grade B)* [4], but few studies are available and optimal dosing schedule in patients with morbid obesty is yet to be determined..

Regional Techniques

Utilizing regional anesthesia to block peripheral or central nerves is an effective option to reduce or eliminate the need for opioids. A continuous infusion of local anesthetics should be considered in patients requiring prolonged analgesia, who are at risk of local anesthetic overdose, and in whom motor function needs to be preserved, like patients undergoing lower extremity joint replacement. Other benefits of continuous nerve block include reduction in hospital resource utilization, decreased risk of nausea and vomiting, early discharge, and improvement in patient satisfaction.

Neuroaxial Techniques

Neuroaxial techniques for pain management have been shown in numerous studies to be highly efficient in reducing opioid-related complications.

Thoracic Epidural Analgesia (TEA)

(T6-T11) remains the gold standard for postoperative pain control in patients undergoing open abdominal surgery. Initiation of neuroaxial blockade before surgery and its maintenance throughout surgical intervention decreases the need for anaesthetic agents, opioids and muscle relaxants [3]. Continuation of regional anesthesia techniques into the postoperative period to provide analgesia is regarded particular useful in obese patients undergoing open bariatric surgery. Compared with parenteral opioids, epidural blockade has shown to provide better postoperative static and dynamic analgesia for the first 72 h, to accelerate the recovery of gastrointestinal function, to reduce insulin resistance and impact positively on cardiovascular and respiratory complications [3]. Epidural analgesia in patients submit to open bariatric surgery resulted in better pain scores, patient satisfaction, early recovery and ambulation *(Recommendation Grade B)* [4]. The same benefits have not been observed after laparoscopic procedures, especially in a context of an ERAS programme. However, TEA might still be valuable in patients at risk of respiratory complications, in those with high probability of conversion to laparotomy, or requiring transverse or Pfannenstiel-like incisions [3].

Intrathecal (IT) Analgesia

IT morphine is a valuable analgesic technique to improve early postoperative analgesia and facilitates surgical recovery. However, compared with systemic opioids, the incidence of pruritus and respiratory depression (although rare) is increased. Postoperative urinary retention is also more frecuent. In the light of these side effects, in the context of an multimodal analgesic regimen other regional anaesthesia technique could be favoured [3].

TAP Blocks

Transvesus abdominis plane (TAP) block has been studied as a potential technique to aid with pain management in bariatric surgery. Field blocks are non-specific, and the local anesthetic mixture is administered in fascial planes between muscles. It has been shown to reduce morphine use and PONV in abdominal surgery *(Recommendation Grade C, especially laparoscopic procedures)* [4]. Other studies have found limited or no statistically significant difference in outcomes with this block. One potential explanation may be that, there is no significant added benefit of TAP block if local anesthetic is also infiltrated at trocar insertion sites. Like all regional techniques, the efficacy of TAP block is also operator dependent, and in patients with morbidly obesity the performance of TAP blocks may be more difficult. However, TAP blocks can also be performed by surgeons from the peritoneal cavity before closing the abdominal wall, or laparoscopic guided.

Intraperitoneal and Wound Modalities

Continuous administration of local anesthetic has been reported at wound and/or intraperitoneal infusions.

Some studies that examines the use of continuos bupivacaine wound infusion in laparoscopic weight loss surgery (WLS) lasting up to 96 hours. There was a statistically significant decrease in opioid consumption, but this benefit was not sustained beyond the infusion and there was no improvement in patient pain scores.

On the other hand, intraperitoneal bupivacaine infusions have found a statistically improvement in pain scores and total opioid consumption. Likewise, the use of a one-time spray of bupivacaine applied at the esophagueal hiatus once the pneumoperitoneum is establish, resulted in statistically significant decreased in analgesic consumption, incluiding shoulder tip pain. For this reasons, these loco-regional analgesic modalities contribute to optimizing pain in open abdominal and laparoscopic surgical procedures (Recommendation Grade C). Further investigations, standardization and technique refinement are required [4].

Conclusion

A multimodal analgesia regimen should de used in patients undergoing open and laparoscopic abdominal procedures with the aim to reduce opioid consumption and their dose-dependent side effects that impair recovery. Analgesic techniques should aim to not only provide optimal pain control, but also to facilitate the achievement of important milestones such as early mobilization. This is of particular importance in this patient population because of the risks of airway obstruction and respiratory insufficiency, otherwise inherent to an opioid centric acute pain management protocols. Opioid-sparing analgesic strategies, including regional analgesia techniques, should be implemented in a context of a multimodal analgesic regimen [3].

REFERENCES

[1] Mauermann E, Ruppen W, Bandschapp O. Different protocols used today to achieve total opioid-free general anesthesia without locoregional blocks. *Best Pract Res Clin Anaesthesiol* 2017; doi: 10.1016/j.bpa.2017.11.003.

[2] Schung SA, Rayman A. Posoperative pain management of the obese patient. *Best Pract Res Clin Anaesthesiol* 2011; 25:73-81.

[3] Feldheiser A, Aziz O, Baldini G, et al. Enhanced Recovery after Surgery (ERAS) for gastrointestinal surgery, part 2: consensus statement for anaesthesia practice. *Acta Anaesthesiol Scand* 2016; 60:289-334.

[4] Budiansky AS, Margarson MP. Acute pain management in morbid obesity- an evidence based clinical update. *Surg Obes Relat Dis* 2017; 13:523-532.

[5] Smetana GW. Postoperative pulmonary complications: an update on risk assessment and reduction. *Cleve Clin J Med* 2009; 76(4):60–S65.

[6] American Society of Anesthesiologists. Practice guidelines for the perioperative management of patients with obstructive sleep apnea. *Anesthesiology* 2006; 104:1081-1093.

[7] Wardhan R, Chelly J. Recent advances in acute pain management: understanding the mechanisms of acute pain, the prescription of opioids, and the role of multimodal pain therapy. *F1000Res* 2017; 6:2065 (doi: 10.12688/f1000research.12286.1).

[8] Schumann R, Jones SB, Cooper B, et al. Update on best practce recommendations for anesthesic perioperative care and pain management in weight loss surgery, 2004-2007. *Obesity* 2009; 17:889-894.

[9] American Society of Anesthesiologists Task Force on Acute Pain Management: Practice guidelines for acute pain management in the perioperative setting: an updated report by the American Society of Anesthesiologists Task Force on Acute Pain Management. *Anesthesiology* 2012; 116(2):248–73.

[10] Wang L, Johnston B, Kaushal A, et al. Ketamine added to morphine or hydromorphone patient-controlled analgesia for acute post-operative pain in adults: a systematic review and meta-analysis of randomized trials. *Can J Anaesth* 2016; 63(3):311–25.

[11] Buvanendran A, Kroin JS. Multimodal analgesia for controlling acute postoperative pain. *Curr Opin anaesthesiol* 2009; 22:588–593.

[12] Tonner PH. Additives used to reduce perioperative opioid consumption1: Alpha2-agonists. *Best Pract Res Clin Anaesthesiol* 2017; doi: 10.1016/j.bpa.2017.10.004.

[13] Estebe JP. Intravenous lidocaine. *Best Pract Res Clin Anaesthesiol* 2017; doi: 10.1016/j.bpa.2017.05.005.

In: Management of Postoperative Pain … ISBN: 978-1-53614-284-6
Editor: Jaime Ruiz-Tovar

Chapter 4

OPIOID FREE ANESTHESIA

Irene Portero, MD*
Department of Anesthesiology, Rey Juan Carlos Hospital, Madrid, Spain

ABSTRACT

Opioid related side effects are numerous. Some of them are potentially dangerous and responsible for important morbidity in post-operative period. Morbidly obese patients are especially at risk due to their changes in respiratory physiology, anatomy, and even sensitivity to opioids. Patients with obstructive sleep apnea present even more risk. Each year, several reasons are added for reducing or avoiding the use of synthetic opioids. Enhanced postoperative recovery may be achieved by reducing opioid use to improve healing and to avoid immune system suppression. If no opioids are used during surgery, fewer opioids are needed to achieve a pain-free recovery.

Keywords: opioid, tolerance, hyperalgesia, recovery

* Corresponding Author: Irene Portero, MD. Email: irene.portero@hospitalreyjuancarlos.es.

Introduction

Before the introduction of opioids, hypnosis, immobility, and hemodynamic stability were achieved using deep inhalational or high-dose hypnotics. These agents also induced strong hemodynamic suppression. Therefore, the introduction of balanced anesthesia was a gift. Opioids support hemodynamic stability by suppressing the sympathetic system. In addition, opioids are the strongest analgesics, and analgesia then came to be an essential part of balanced anesthesia, together with hypnosis and immobility.

20 years ago it was already known that short-acting opioids could cause addiction, immunosuppression, and other unknown long-term effects, and that high-dose opioids are not needed to achieve anesthesia. Nevertheless, anesthesiologists were drawn to the use of these powerful opioids due to their seemingly short activity. Moreover, the combination of opioids and new low-dose intravenous hypnotics such as propofol, without inhalational agents, became attractive to suppress postoperative nausea and vomiting and retain hemodynamic stability. Side effects of the inhalational agents were avoided, but are the side effects of opioids not more dramatic and prolonged?

Most common side effects of opioids are well known: respiratory depression, pruritus, nausea and vomiting, ileus, constipation, urinary retention, tolerance by desensitization, immediate hyperalgesia that may evolve into chronic pain syndrome, reduced cardiac output, dizziness, somnolence, and short-duration central muscle stiffness.

Opioid-induced ventilatory impairment is well known by anesthesiologists and easily treated in the post-anesthesia care unit, but this complication is still problematic postoperatively on the ward.

A lesser known side effect is pharyngeal muscle weakness, contributing to obstructive breathing patterns in every patient. This side effect should certainly be avoided in obese patients and patients with obstructive sleep apnea (OSA), given the potential for aggravation and further breathing obstruction. Accordingly, recommendations for anesthesiologists are to avoid or minimize the perioperative use of opioids in these patients.

In addition to their side effects, the addition of, abuse of and tolerance to opioids have become a major problem.

Two famous publications in the 80's, one a letter to the editor purporting that addiction was rare in patients treated with opioids, and the other, a retrospective analysis demonstrating the safety of opioids in 38 chronic pain patients, opened the flood gates to opioid prescription writing from the 1990s to the 2000s. These two publications were used in intense marketing efforts by pharmaceutical companies to convince physicians that opioids could be used safely in treating acute and chronic pain. The dangers associated with opioids, namely their high abuse potential and lethality when taken in excess or in combination with other drugs, were often downplayed. Multiple studies documented a strong and consistent linear relationship between the increase in pain assessment, the volume of opioid sales for treatment, and the morbidity and mortality associated with these products. Non-medical use of prescription opioids is now one of the most serious public health problems in the United States, and has resulted in unprecedented rates of accidental death and opioid-related treatment admissions. Drug overdose death rates in the United States increased 5-fold between 1980 and 2008, mirroring the introduction of the fifth vital sign and making drug overdose a leading cause of injury and death. Up to 8% of opioid-naive patients who undergo surgery and receive opioids perioperatively may become chronic opioid users. Each year several reasons are added for reducing or avoiding the use of synthetic opioids. Enhanced postoperative recovery may be achieved by reducing opioid use to improve healing and to avoid immune system suppression.

When Do We Need Opioids?

The absence of pain is only needed postoperatively when patients are awake. Perioperatively, we need a stress-free anesthesia to achieve hemodynamic and general physiological stability.

We have to guarantee sufficient tissue perfusion to provide nutrients and oxygen and to remove carbon dioxide and waste. Opioids were the ideal agents to address these needs in the past, but today it is possible to block sympathetic reactions and achieve hemodynamic stability with other drugs.

Over the past years, more and more studies have found that patient outcomes also improve without opioids.

The higher doses of opioids following surgery were associated with an increased length of stay (LOS). And the more opioids you give intraoperatively, the more you will need postoperatively.

This new approach in anesthesia provides hypnosis with amnesia and muscle relaxation, if needed, while ensures sufficient tissue perfusion and sympathetic stability to protect organs avoiding opioids. In the past, hypnotics available were important cardiovascular depressants, high doses of opioids allowed the reduction of hypnotics and muscle relaxants leading to a better hemodynamic control.

Opioids and Respiratory Failure

It is well known that all opioids agonists produce respiratory depression via effects on mu and delta receptors in respiratory center. They also reduce responsiveness of the respiratory center to increasing carbon dioxide and decreasing oxygen levels.

But opioid receptors are also found on mechanosensory receptors in the airways. They activate laryngeal adductor motor neurons and depress laryngeal abductor and pharyngeal constrictor motor neurons, thereby decreasing upper airway diameter.

Opioids increase upper airway obstruction in every patient; whether this would be clinically relevant or not, would depend on other factors such as obesity. Other anesthetics, like propofol and midazolam, induce and aggravate upper airway obstruction, when combined with opioids. Only ketamine and dexmedetomidine seem to have minimal effects on upper airway diameter.

Opioid Tolerance

Long-term use of opioids can be problematic because of the rapid development of tolerance to the analgesic effects coupled with the slow development of tolerance to many of the side-effects.

Acute tolerance is mediated predominantly by pharmacodynamic mechanisms, manifested as a decreased response following a single administration of the agent. Acute pharmacodynamic tolerance occurs when the response of the receptor diminishes over time; therefore, any ability to reduce opioid use post-operatively without avoiding intra-operative opioids will fail.

Opioid Induced Hyperalgesia

It is defined as a state of nociceptive sensitization caused by exposure to opioids. The condition is characterized by a paradoxical response whereby a patient receiving opioids for the treatment of pain might actually become more sensitive to certain painful stimuli.

Opioid reinforcement of central sensitization in inflammatory pain states could be partially prevented by small amounts of N-methyl-D-aspartate receptor blockers like ketamine. Therefore, ketamine at doses of 0.25 mg/kg might be clinically useful in OSAS patients if opioids cannot be excluded perioperatively. At this dose, ketamine has some analgesic properties and limited hallucination effects.

Opioids induce or aggravate obstructive breathing in all patients, including patients with OSAS. Therefore, it was thought that short-acting opioids like remifentanil would be ideal for OSAS patients. However, the increased postoperative pain because of central sensitization by remifentanil requires additional opioid treatment, which increases the risk.

It is important to identify methods to reduce the need for intra-operative opioid use, which then will facilitate the reduction of postoperative opioid use.

One option is to use loco-regional anesthesia alone or in combination with general anesthesia based on hypnotics without opioids.

A second approach is to avoid all opioids during general anesthesia by relying on hypnotics to induce sleep and use drugs that block the autonomic nervous system reaction to pain stimuli.

The approach of using opioid-free anesthesia combined with multimodal postoperative analgesia, reduces the need for more additional therapy post- operatively in OSAS patients.

INDICATIONS AND CONTRAINDICATIONS

The following are the general indications and contraindications for Opioid Free Anesthesia techniques.

Indications

- Narcotic abuse history (acute or chronic opioid addiction);
- Opioid intolerance;
- Morbidity obese patients with obstructive sleep apnea
- Hyperalgesia;
- History of chronic pain, immune deficiency, oncologic surgery or inflammatory diseases;
- History of postoperative nausea and vomiting;
- High risk of postoperative pulmonary morbidity;
- Enhanced recovery After Surgery protocols.

Contraindications

Absolute

- Allergy to any coadjuvant drugs.

Relative

- Disorders of autonomic system;
- Cerebrovascular disease;
- Critical coronary stenosis;
- Extreme bradycardia/block;
- Hypovolemic shock or polytrauma patients;
- Elderly patients on beta-blockers.

OFA IN BARIATRIC SURGERY

Some of the reasons to avoid opioids, besides respiratory depression are: muscle weakness, excessive somnolence, post-operative nausea and vomiting, ileus and constipation, urinary retention, dizziness, obstructive breathing, negative inotropism, and the possibility of tolerance and addiction. Post-operatively, the patient's respiratory system may be too depressed to pass extubation criteria. If able to extubate, early mobilization may be difficult if the patient is too somnolent and experiencing dizziness or PONV, which leads to further complications.

Another important benefit to opioid-free general anesthesia includes the prevention of opioid-induced hyperalgesia, which results in increased pain, thus requiring a higher dose of opioid use to adequately control pain.

Wound healing can also be impaired, which in a population where diabetes is a co-morbidity, can be devastating

These are all valid reasons why opioids should be avoided in bariatric surgery:

1. Avoidance of remifentanil and opioid induced hyperalgesia;
2. OSA and other opioid mediated problems eliminated;
3. Easily "protocol-driven";
4. Aids optimization of "laparoscopic working space";
5. Guarantees analgesia and sympathetic blockade/moderate amnesia;
6. Awareness unlikely if BIS (entropy) is kept below 60.

Mulier's opioid-free technique has been referred to as the MuliMix, where one to three of the following techniques are used:

1. Sympatholysis, analgesia, and anesthesia (MAC reduction) with dexmedetomidine;
2. Analgesia with low-dose ketamine;
3. Co-anesthesia and sympatholysis with intravenous lidocaine;
4. Profound neuromuscular blockade maintained up to the end of surgery and appropriately reversed;
5. 0.7 -1.0 MAC desflurane in oxygen/air titrated to entropy or BIS EEG monitoring;
6. Magnesium infusion as a further co-analgesic.

The research into non-opioid anesthesia has brought dexmedetomidine, ketamine, lidocaine, magnesium, clonidine, and ketorolac into the forefront as alternative non-opioid anesthesia adjuncts. The mechanism of action of these adjuncts differs from one another, thus providing pain management by targeting multiple sites in the pain pathway. The ideal combination of these adjuncts may not be perfected at this time, but understanding the mechanism of action helps the anesthesia provider utilize such drugs to their full potential.

A recent systematic analysis on opioid free general anesthesia versus opioid based general anesthesia in bariatric surgery concludes that post-operative pain management can be reached without any or a reduced amount of opioids, but without the opioid side effects. This aids in less PONV episodes and less complications from surgery, which can result in a decrease in length of stay in the PACU. The latter can be debated, as some studies have shown no statistical significance in the length of recovery in the PACU between opioid-free general anesthesia and opioid-based general anesthesia. It seems fair to extrapolate that less complications will result in less time spent in the PACU.

Obviously, we should not forget contraindications and be aware that there are some disadvantages, such as:

1. Ketamine perturbs the EEG monitoring of awareness.
2. Some patients will require vasopressor support.
3. OFA may have to be breached to achieve ideal intubating conditions with small doses of short acting opioid.
4. Cutaneous vasoconstriction - an expected alpha 2 effect may alarm clinicians.
5. There is clearly a learning curve for the individual and institution.
6. Awareness is a possibility if the technique is incorrectly applied or misused.

Understanding the pathophysiology of the obese patients is imperative, but moving forward, improving the safety of anesthesia provided to this unique population needs to be further addressed. Using existing research, medications such as dexmedetomidine, ketamine, lidocaine, magnesium, and ketorolac have shown to be effective pain management alternatives to opioids.

Anesthesia providers, such as Mulier and Sultana, extrapolated these results into bariatric surgery and reported better postoperative outcomes. The literature review indicates that pain in the obese patient can be managed with an opioid-free anesthetic plan, while avoiding opioid-induced complications.

Opioid-free anesthesia might be the solution and the future of anesthesia management of the obese patient undergoing bariatric surgery, but more evidence- based research is needed in order to change the practice of anesthesia.

References

Ahmad S, Nagle A, McCarthy RJ, et al. Postoperative hypoxemia in morbidly obese patients with and without obstructive sleep apnea undergoing laparoscopic bariatric surgery. *Anesth Analg* 2008; 107:138–143

Bernards CM, Knowlton S, Schmidt D, et al. Respiratory and sleep effects of remifentanil in volunteers with moderate obstructive sleep apnea. *Anesthesiology* 2009; 110:41–49.

Duarte LTD, Fernandes MCBC, Costa VV, et al. The incidence of post-operative respiratory depression in patients undergoing intravenous or epidural analgesia with opioids. *Rev Bras Anestesiol* 2009; 59:409–420.

Ehsan Z, Mahmoud M, Shott SR, et al. *The effects of anesthesia and opioids on the upper airway: a systematic review.* Laryngoscope 2015.

Feld JM, Laurito CE, Beckerman M, et al. Nonopioid analgesia improves pain relief and decreases sedation after gastric bypass surgery. *Can J Anaesth* 2003; 50:336 – 341.

Fletcher D, Martinez V. Opioid-induced hyperalgesia in patients after surgery: a systematic review and a meta-analysis. *British Journal of Anaesthesia* 2014; 112(6): 991–1004.

Funk RD, Hilliard P, Ramachandran SK. Perioperative Opioid Usage: Avoiding Adverse Effects. *Plast. Reconstr. Surg.* 2014; 134: 32S.

Isono S. Obesity and obstructive sleep apnoea: Mechanisms for increased collapsibility of the passive pharyngeal airway. *Respirology.* 2012;17:32-42.

Mason M, Cates CJ, Smith I. Effects of opioid, hypnotic and sedating medications on sleep-disordered breathing in adults with obstructive sleep apnoea. *Cochrane Database Syst Rev* 2015; 14:7.

Mulier J, Dillemans B, Van Lancker P. Opioid free (OFA) versus opioid (OA) and low opioid anesthesia (LOA) for the laparoscopic gastric bypass surgery. Immediate post operative morbidity and mortality in a single center study on 5061 consecutive patients from March 2011 till June 2015. *Eur J Anesthesiology* 2016; 33(e-S54):90.

Randerath WJ, George S. Opioid-induced sleep apnea: is it a real problem? *J Clin Sleep Med* 2012; 8:577–578.

Said Q, Evans R, Gregory J, Stoddard G, Lloyd J, Jackson K et al. Opioid-Related Adverse Drug Events in Surgical Hospitalizations: Impact on Costs and Length of Stay. *The Annals of Pharmacotherapy.* 2007;41(3):400-407.

Umutoglu T, Topuz U, Uysal H, Bayram M, Kadioglu H et al. Opioid-free total intravenous anesthesia with propofol, dexmedetomidine and lidocaine infusions for laparoscopic cholecystectomy: a prospective, randomized, double-blinded study. *Rev Bras Anestesiol.* 2015; 65(3):191-199.

Weinbroum A. Role of anaesthetics and opioids in perioperative hyperalgesia. *Eur J Anaesthesiol* 2015; 32:230–231.

White PF. The changing role of non-opioid analgesic techniques in the management of postoperative pain. *Anesth Analg* 2005; 101:S5–S22.

In: Management of Postoperative Pain ... ISBN: 978-1-53614-284-6
Editor: Jaime Ruiz-Tovar

Chapter 5

IMPLICATIONS OF LAPAROSCOPIC APPROACH ON POSTOPERATIVE PAIN AFTER BARIATRIC SURGERY

Pablo Priego**, MD, PhD
Department of General Surgery,
Division of Esophagogastric and Bariatric Surgery,
Ramón y Cajal University Hospital, Madrid, Spain

ABSTRACT

Laparoscopy has shown to have special benefits to obese patients because of less blood loss, earlier mobilization, reduced postoperative pain, shorter hospital stay and faster convalescence in comparison with the open procedure. Moreover, the risk of intraabdominal adhesions and incisional hernia has cleared decreased. Pain management is a significant component of postoperative care. The traumatic effect of the surgical incision, the mobilization of intraabdominal viscera during surgery, and some of the metabolic responses that accompany surgery are the main responsible in the occurrence of postoperative pain and complications. Implications of laparoscopic approach against open procedure on postoperative pain after bariatric surgery are presented in this chapter.

* Corresponding Author Email: papriego@hotmail.com.

Keywords: open, laparoscopy, bariatric surgery, postoperative pain, analgesia, gastric bypass

INTRODUCTION

The number of bariatric procedures has recently risen up, not only because an increase of the number of obese patients, but also because of the exponential growth up in the number of laparoscopic surgeries performed. In USA, Nguyen et al., [1] using NIS data estimated that the percentage of bariatric procedures performed laparoscopically increased from 2.1% in 1998 to 17.9% in 2002. Nowadays, it is not very common to perform a bariatric surgery through an open approach.

Laparoscopy has shown to have special benefits to obese patients because of less blood loss, earlier mobilization, reduced postoperative pain, shorter hospital stay and faster convalescence in comparison with the open procedure. Moreover, the risk of intraabdominal adhesions and incisional hernia has clearly decreased [2].

However, when comparing the outcomes of a bariatric operation performed by two different approaches, it is essential to choose which outcome measures are determinant for clinical practice. Nguyen et al., [3], argue that sometimes, the most common measurements outcome include operative time and length of hospital stay. Furthermore, and although a short surgical time is preferred, this is not always correlated with a better operative outcome. In the same way, the hospital stay can be misleading because it only represents the time of hospitalization that it is considered to be safe before a patient is discharge home. For these reasons, these two parameters would not be as good enough in order to show the superiority to one technique over the other. From the patient's view better measures will be the postoperative pain and duration of the convalescence.

Pain management is a significant component of postoperative care. The traumatic effect of the surgical incision, the mobilization of intraabdominal viscera during surgery, and some of the metabolic responses that accompany surgery are the main responsible in the occurrence of postoperative pain. Moreover, postoperative pain may also be a pointer to the development of certain complications like atelectasia, pneumonia, deep vein thrombosis, pulmonary embolism and cardio-vascular events [4].

Implications of laparoscopic approach against open procedure on postoperative pain after bariatric surgery are presented in this chapter.

Open vs. Laparoscopic Bariatric Surgery

Since the introduction of laparoscopic surgery, a wide variety of techniques have been performed via this approach because of the advantages it offers, i.e., earlier mobilization, reduced postoperative pain, shorter hospital stay, better cosmetic results and faster convalescence in comparison with the open procedure. Moreover, the risk of intraabdominal adhesions and incisional hernia has clearly decreased [2].

Therefore, surgeons began using the different techniques that existed for treating obesity through the laparoscopic approach [5, 6]. *Gastric banding* was the first laparoscopic technique described which became extremely popular due to its relatively low technical difficulty and low initial morbidity and mortality rates [7-9]. However, long-term results regarding weight loss and late complications were worse than with other bariatric procedures.

Another of the procedures performed via laparoscopy was *Vertical banded gastroplasty* [10, 11]. This technique was not difficult to perform by laparoscopy and had low morbidity and mortality rates, but the long-term results were worse than with gastric bypass and nowadays it is not a common option for treatment of obese patients, due to the discomfort it causes the patient and the high incidence of staple-line disruption.

Gastric bypass (GB) was initially developed in USA by Masson and Ito in the 1960s [12]. Although GB resulted in durable weight loss and had evident advantages like better weight loss than after purely restrictive procedures, low incidence of protein-calorie malnutrition, rapid improvement of resolution of weigh-related comorbidities and appetite reduction; postoperative pain and wound-related complications such as infection (8%) and incisional hernia (20%) were disgusting problems.

Laparoscopic gastric bypass (LGBP) was first introduced by Wittgrove et al., [13] in 1994 and since then has become more commonly performed than open gastric bypass (OGB).

Although there are several restrictive (gastric band, sleeve gastrectomy) and malabsortive weight loss operations (duodenal switch, SADI-s, biliopancreatic diversion…), most of studies comparing open vs. laparoscopic approach are related to GB, because nowadays it is the most common bariatric procedure all around the world.

From the beginning, clinical studies [6, 14, 15] demonstrated that LGBP was a safe and effective alternative to OGB for the treatment of morbid obesity. Moreover, laparoscopy showed a lot of advantages against the traditional open approach. On the other hand, LGBP showed that this was a complex operation associated with a long learning curve and with a possible increase in the rate of internal hernia [16-18].

Most part of studies that compare open vs. laparoscopy in bariatric surgery are too old (final of the 90s and beginning of 21st century), because nowadays, there is not discussion about the advantages of this minimally invasive approach in the treatment of these obese patients. Indeed, current studies are concerning about differences in postoperative pain and cosmetic results between the single-port and the traditional laparoscopic approach [19, 20]. Other studies present that the implementation of Enhanced Recovery After Surgery (ERAS) programs [21] in treatment of obese patients is a safe issue, obtaining similar results to standard care in terms of complications, reoperations, mortality and readmissions; with less postoperative pain and earlier hospital discharge. Other studies are referred to the decrease of postoperative pain associated with the intraoperative peritoneal infusion with ropivacaine [22] and the postoperative advantages of free opioids anesthesia [23]. However, these items have been described in other chapters of the book.

In order to understand differences between open and laparoscopic approach in bariatric surgery, it is essential to differentiate some technical aspects that are going to affect clinical outcomes [3].

The first difference between these two approaches is the method of access (length and number of abdominal incisions). OGB is usually performed through a supraumbilical midline incision, whereas LGBP is performed through five-six small abdominal incisions for trocars.

Second difference is the method of exposure. During OGB, the methods of exposure are abdominal wall retractors and mechanical retractors of intraabdominal organs. On the other hand, in LGBP, methods of exposure are the pneumoperitoneum to create a working space and gravity for moving of intraabdominal organs.

Finally, the last difference is the extent of operative trauma. By reducing the length of the surgical incision and avoiding the needed of abdominal wall retractors, it is logical that operative trauma is less in after LGBP in compare to OGB.

Although physiopathological basis of postoperative pain have been presented in Chapter 1, we cannot avoid that there are some physiopathological differences between open and laparoscopic surgery that influences in the development of postoperative pain.

Surgical injury often results in accumulation of edema (third-space fluid), and the degree of third-space fluid accumulation is often proportional to the extent of surgical trauma. Indeed, intra-abdominal pressure after LGBP is significantly lower than after OGB on postoperative days 1, 2, and 3. Moreover, the magnitude of the systemic stress response (interleukin-6 levels) is significantly lower after LGBP than after OGB.

Providing a high quality pain treatment is a major challenge in health care. Despite the developments in pain management, postoperative pain is still a clinical problem [24-26]. Poorly managed pain reduces quality of life, causes unneeded suffering, and can extend time of discharge from hospital [27]. The importance of evaluating postoperative pain with consideration given to type of surgery and the patient's perspective cannot be overemphasized. Postoperative pain is an important measurement of outcome because it can be measured objectively. The degree of postoperative pain after OGB is associated with the length of the surgical incision, the extent of operative dissection, and operative trauma [26].

Hence, laparoscopic procedures that minimize surgical tissue trauma are associated with less pain than laparotomies [29-30].

While some outcomes such as pulmonary complications, duration of hospital stay and convalescence appear to be better with the laparoscopic approach [31, 32], few prospective trials have investigated the effect of LGBP on postoperative pain and bowel function.

One of the first studies that compare open vs. laparoscopic approach in bariatric surgery was the study of Joris et al., [33]. They compared a group of 30 obese patients undergoing laparoscopic or open gastroplasty (15 in each group). Postoperative pain, measured on a visual analogue scale (VAS), and opioid consumption were recorded during the first two days after operation. Tests of pulmonary function were performed and SpO2 was measured 4 h after surgery and on days 1, 2 and 3 after operation. Results confirmed that in the laparoscopy group, requirements for postoperative opioid were 50% less; pain intensity during mobilization and on coughing was significantly less after laparoscopy. Forced vital capacity, forced expiratory volume in 1 s and peak expiratory flow rate were reduced significantly less after laparoscopic gastroplasty than after open gastroplasty. Moreover, SpO_2 values were significantly greater in the laparoscopy group.

El Shoraby et al., [34], performed a prospective study in which patients were assigned to LGBP (33 cases) or OGB (20 cases). All patients received patient controlled analgesia (PCA) with intravenous morphine and rectal naproxen 500 mg every 12 hours. Postoperative analgesia was assessed daily using a VAS at rest, on walking and coughing. The amount of morphine used during the first 48 hours, the time of return of gastrointestinal motility and the time until first oral food intake were recorded. Patients undergoing LGBP requested less morphine and showed lower VAS pain scores than patients undergoing OGB. The return of bowel movement in the laparoscopic group occurred 1 day earlier than in the open group. The time to first passage of gas and oral food intake was shorter after laparoscopic than after OGB. Moreover, patients in the laparoscopic group were discharged 1.5 days earlier than patients in the open group.

Fisher [35] randomly selected bariatric surgery patients, consisting of 20 OGB, 19 LGBP, and 21 laparoscopic adjustable gastric banding (LAGB). LAGB patients returned to normal activity levels earlier than gastric bypass patient's irrespective of approach. Moreover, recovering from surgery was significantly sooner than OGB patients. However, perceived differences in recovery time between OGB and LGBP patients did not affect their time to resumption of normal activity.

Finally, Nguyen et al., [3] performed a randomized study in which seventy obese patients were randomly assigned to undergo LGBP (n = 36) or OGB (n = 34). Pulmonary function studies were performed preoperatively and on postoperative days 1, 2, 3, and 7. Oxygen saturation and chest radiographs were performed on both groups preoperatively and on postoperative day 1. Postoperative pain was evaluated using a VAS and the amount of narcotic consumed was recorded. LGBP patients had significantly less impairment of pulmonary function than OGB patients on the first three postoperative days. By the 7th postoperative day, all pulmonary function parameters in the LGBP group had returned to within preoperative levels, but only one parameter (peak expiratory flow) had returned to preoperative levels in the OGB group. Moreover, on the first postoperative day, LGBP patients used less intravenous morphine sulfate than OGB patients (46 +/- 31 mg versus 76 +/- 39 mg, respectively), and VAS pain scores at rest and during mobilization were lower after LGBP than after OGB. Fewer patients after LGBP than after OGB developed hypoxemia (31% versus 76%) and segmental atelectasia (6% versus 55%). All results were statistically significant.

Recovery is a very important outcome parameter and can be measured by questioning the patients' time to return to activities of daily living. Nguyen et al., [15] reported that LGBP patients had a more rapid return to activities of daily living than OGB patients. Furthermore, and based on the SF-36 health survey and the Moorehead-Ardelt Quality-of-Life questionnaire it has shown that recovery based on physical and social functioning at 1 and 3 months postoperatively was significantly faster after LGBP compared to OGB. In addition, patients undergoing laparoscopic surgery perceived their overall health to be better than that of OGB patients when the survey was measured at 1 month postoperatively. Moreover, LGBP patients had more sexual interest or resumed sexual activity earlier than OGB patients at 3 months postoperatively, hence demonstrating a faster recovery.

However, and although LGBP is considered as a minimally invasive procedure, most of the patients complain of abdominal pain after surgery [36-38]. Cho et al., [36], have reported that 98.94% of patients were found to have pain in the first 24 hours of post-surgery, 60% at the end of the first week and 29.5% still had pain four weeks after the surgery. The highest incidence of abdominal pain was in left upper quadrant. Moreover, 45% of patients were admitted to the emergency department complaining of abdominal pain. About 54.1% of these patients were referred again for the second time and 22.6% were admitted for the third time, all due to abdominal pain.

Eidy et al., [39], analyzed the distribution and frequency of post LGBP pain in 190 morbidly obese patients. The results of the study were similar to those published by Cho et al., Left upper quadrant was found to be the most prevalent site for pain, probably related to the insertion of drainage.

There are many reasons for pain after gastric bypass surgeries, several of which could be related to the behavioral eating patterns, such as rapid eating [40], food intolerance, like rice, vegetables, fruits, pasta, gluten and lactose intolerance, some deficiencies like folate and vitamin B12 deficiencies [41] and finally bacterial overgrowth [42]. Other etiologies could be constipation and lower abdominal pain due functional changes of the gastrointestinal tract after surgery, retroesternal pain, biliar colics because of de novo gallbladder stones, ulcers in gastric pouch, gastroesophageal reflux disease (GERD), anastomotic stenosis, trocar site hernia, adhesions band, incisional hernia, intussusceptions, omental torsion, infarction, internal hernia and bezoars.

Similar to other minimal invasive operations, the late pain following GB surgery is a serious problem. Chronic postsurgical pain (CPSP) has been defined as pain persisting for more than 3 months after expected healing time. CPSP of the surgical site after bariatric surgery has been reported in up to 50% of the patients.

Finally, Kumar et al., [4], performed a review of the literature in order to identify follow-up studies on pain and bariatric surgery. Sixteen studies were included for further analysis with over 2000 subjects (60% of them were on bypass surgery). "Short term" studies with data on pain within 3 months after surgery were randomized controlled trials comparing surgical techniques or analgesia. Although pre-operative pain status had not been documented, peri-operative pain management was reported in detail. In 8 observational studies, pain data were available exceeding 3 months after surgery ("long term" studies). While pre-operative pain data were reported in the latter studies, in over half the anatomic location of the pain had not been specified. Authors concluded that an accurate estimation of the incidence of CPSP after bariatric surgery was not possible based on the available data. The reason is that number of comparable studies was low and the anatomic location of the pain had not been specified. Moreover, data on pain between 1 week and 6 months after surgery (time point after measured pain is defined as chronic) were lacking.

To end up, the laparoscopic approach has shown to have special benefits to obese patients because of less blood loss, earlier mobilization, reduced postoperative pain, shorter hospital stay and faster convalescence in comparison with the open procedure. Nowadays, there is no discussion about whether laparoscopy should be the treatment of choice for bariatric patients. However, and although laparoscopic gastric bypass is considered as a minimally invasive procedure, many patients complain of abdominal pain after surgery, and chronic postsurgical pain has been reported in up to 50% of the patients. Despite the developments in pain management, postoperative pain is still a clinical problem.

REFERENCES

[1] Nguyen NT, Root J, Zainabadi K, et al., Accelerated growth of bariatric surgery with the introduction of minimally invasive surgery. *Arch Surg*. 2005; 140:1198-1202.

[2] Allvin R, Rawal N, Johanzon E, and Bäckström R. Open versus *Laparoscopic Surgery: Does the Surgical Technique Influence Pain Outcome? Results from an International Registry*. Hindawi Publishing Corporation Pain Research and Treatment. Volume 2016, Article ID 4087325, 5 pages. http://dx.doi.org/10.1155/2016/408 7325.

[3] Nguyen N. Open vs laparoscopic procedures in bariatric surgery. *J Gastrointest Surg* 2004; 8: 393-395.

[4] Kumar N, Soekarman D, Singh R, Bashah MM, Abou Samra AB, Marcus MAE. Peri-operative pain in patients experiencing bariatric surgery. *Med Clin Arch* 2017, 1(1):2-4.

[5] Encinosa WE, Bernard DM, Steiner CA. Advances in bariatric surgery for obesity: laparoscopic surgery. *Adv Health Econ Health Serv Res.* 2007; 17:131-148.

[6] Luján JA, Frutos MD, Hernández Q, et al., Laparoscopic versus open gastric bypass in the treatment of morbid obesity: a randomized prospective study. *Ann Surg*. 2004; 239(4):433-437.

[7] Belachew M, Legrand M, Vincent, et al., Laparoscopic Adjustable gastric banding. *World J Surg* 1998; 22: 955-963.

[8] O'Brien PE, Brown WA, Smith A, et al., Prospective study of a laparoscopically placed, adjustable gastric band in the treatment of morbid obesity. *Br J Surg* 1999; 86: 113-118.

[9] Dargent J. Laparoscopic adjustable gastric banding: lessons from the first 500 patients in a single institution. *Obes Surg* 1999; 9: 446-452.

[10] Hess DW, Hess DS. Laparoscopic vertical banded gastroplasty with complete transection of the staple line. *Obes Surg* 1994; 4: 44-46.

[11] Lönroth H, Dalenbäck J, Haglind E, et al., Vertical banded gastroplasty by laparoscopic technique in the treatment of morbid obesity. *Surg Laparosc Endosc* 1996; 6: 102-107.

[12] Mason EE, Ito C. Gastric bypass in obesity. *Surg Clin North Am.* 1967; 47:1345–1351.

[13] Wittgrove AC, Clark GW, Tremblay LJ. Laparoscopic gastric bypass, Roux-en-Y: preliminary report of five cases. *Obes Surg.* 1994; 4(4):353-357.

[14] Higa KD, Boone KB, Ho T. Complications of the laparoscopic Rouxen-Y gastric bypass: 1,040 patients—what have we learned? *Obesity Surg* 2000; 10:509 –513.

[15] Nguyen NT, Goldman C, Rosenquist CJ, et al., Laparoscopic versus open gastric bypass: a randomized study of outcomes, quality of life, and costs. *Ann Surg*. 2001; 234(3):279-289, discussion 289-291.

[16] Banka G, Woodard G, Hernandez-Boussard T, Morton JM. Laparoscopic vs Open Gastric Bypass Surgery Differences in Patient Demographics, Safety, and Outcomes. *Arch Surg*. 2012; 147(6):550-556.

[17] Weller WE, Rosati C. Comparing outcomes of laparoscopic versus open bariatric surgery. *Ann Surg*. 2008; 248(1):10-15.

[18] Westling A, Gustavsson S. Laparoscopic vs Open Roux –en-Y Gastric Bypass: A prospective, randomized trial. *Obes Surg* 2001; 11: 284-292.

[19] Moreno-Sanz C, Morandeira-Rivas A, Sedano-Vizcaino C, Tenías-Burillo JM, Román-Ortíz C, de la Espada JB. Single-incision laparoscopic bariatric surgery: a systematic review. *Surg Obes Relat Dis*. 2015; 11(1):248-257.

[20] Morales-Conde S, Del Agua IA, Moreno AB, Macías MS. Postoperative pain after conventional laparoscopic versus single-port sleeve gastrectomy: a prospective, randomized, controlled pilot study. *Surg Obes Relat Dis*. 2017; 13(4):608-613.

[21] Ruiz-Tovar J, Muñoz JL, Royo P, Duran M, Redondo E, Ramirez JM; Grupo Español de Rehabilitación Multimodal (GERM). Implementation of the Spanish ERAS program in bariatric surgery. *Minim Invasive Ther Allied Technol*. 2018; 8:1-8.

[22] Ruiz-Tovar J, Gonzalez J, Garcia A, Cruz C, Rivas S, Jimenez M, Ferrigni C, Duran M Intraperitoneal Ropivacaine Irrigation in Patients Undergoing Bariatric Surgery: a Prospective Randomized Clinical Trial. *Obes Surg*. 2016; 26(11):2616-2621.

[23] Barajas JS, Gonzalez D. Pain management in weight loss surgery: aiming for multimodal approach. *Adv Obes Weight Manag Control* 2016, 5(2): 00125.

[24] Benhamou D, Berti M, Brodner G, et al., Postoperative Analgesic THerapy Observational Survey (PATHOS): a practice pattern study in 7 central/southern European countries. *Pain* 2008; 136 (1-2): 134–141.

[25] Hartog CS, Rothaug J, Goettermann A, Zimmer A, and Meissner W. Room for improvement: nurses' and physicians' views of a post-operative pain management program. *Acta Anaesthesiologica Scandinavica* 2010; 54(3):277–283.

[26] Fletcher D, Fermanian C, Mardaye A, Aegerter P. A patient-based national survey on postoperative pain management in France reveals significant achievements and persistent challenges. *Pain* 2008; 137 (2): 441–451.

[27] Taylor RS, Ullrich K, Regan S et al., The impact of early postoperative pain on health-related quality of life. *Pain Practice* 2013; 13 (7): 515–523.

[28] Nguyen NT, Goldman C, Rosenquist CJ, et al., Laparoscopic versus open gastric bypass: a randomized study of outcomes, quality of life, and costs. *Ann Surg*. 2001; 234(3):279-289, discussion 289-291.

[29] Karayiannakis AJ, Makri GG, Mantzioka A, et al., Postoperative pulmonary function after laparoscopic and open cholecystectomy. *Br J Anaesth* 1996; 77:448-452.

[30] Joris J, Cigarini I, Legrand M, et al., Metabolic and respiratory changes after cholecystectomy performed via laparotomy or laparoscopy. *Br J Anaesth* 1992; 69:341-345.

[31] Nguyen N, Lee S, Goldman C, et al., Comparison of pulmonary function and postoperative pain after laparoscopic versus open gastric bypass: a randomized trial. *J Am Coll Surg* 2001; 192: 469-476; discussion 476-477.

[32] Antoniou SA, Antoniou GA, Koch OO, Köhler G, Pointner R, Granderath FA. Laparoscopic versus Open Obesity Surgery: A Meta-Analysis of Pulmonary Complications. *Dig Surg* 2015; 32:98–107.

[33] Joris JL, Hinque VL, Laurent PE, et al., Pulmonary function and pain after gastroplasty performed via laparotomy or laparoscopy in morbidly obese patients. *Br J Anaesth* 1998; 80: 283-288.

[34] El Shobary H, Christou N, Backman SB, Gvocdic B, Schricker T. Effect of Laparoscopic versus Open Gastric Bypass Surgery on Postoperative Pain and Bowel Function. *Obes Surg* 2006; 16:437-442.

[35] Fisher BL. Comparison of recovery time after open and laparoscopic gastric bypass and laparoscopic adjustable banding. *Obes Surg*. 2004; 14(1):67-72.

[36] Cho M, Kaidar-Person O, Szomstein S, Rosenthal RJ. Emergency room visits after laparoscopic Roux-en-Y gastric bypass for morbid obesity. *Surg Obes Relat Dis.* 2008; 4(2):104–109.

[37] Kellogg TA, Swan T, Leslie DA, Buchwald H, Ikramuddin S. Patterns of readmission and reoperation within 90 days after Roux-en-Y gastric bypass. *Surg Obes Relat Dis.* 2009; 5(4):416–423.

[38] Agaba EA, Gentles CV, Shamseddeen H, Sasthakonar V, Kandel A, Gadelata D, et al., Retrospective analysis of abdominal pain in postoperative laparoscopic Roux-en-Y gastric bypass patients: is a simple algorithm the answer? *Surg Obes Relat Dis.* 2008; 4(5): 587–593.

[39] Eidy M, Pazouki A, Raygan F, Ariyazand Y, Pishgahroudsari M, Jesmi F. Functional abdominal pain syndrome in morbidly obese patients following laparoscopic gastric bypass surgery. *Arch Trauma Res*. 2014 Mar 20; 3(1):e13110.

[40] Foster A, Richards WO, McDowell J, Laws HL, Clements RH. Gastrointestinal symptoms are more intense in morbidly obese patients. *Surg Endosc.* 2003; 17(11):1766–1768.

[41] Walker SP, Wein P, Ihle BU. Severe folate deficiency masquerading as the syndrome of hemolysis, elevated liver enzymes, and low platelets. *Obstet Gynecol.* 1997; 90 (4 Pt 2):655–657.

[42] Ishida RK, Faintuch J, Paula AM, Risttori CA, Silva SN, Gomes ES, et al., Microbial flora of the stomach after gastric bypass for morbid obesity. *Obes Surg*. 2007; 17(6):752–758.

In: Management of Postoperative Pain ... ISBN: 978-1-53614-284-6
Editor: Jaime Ruiz-Tovar

Chapter 6

PORT SITE INFILTRATION WITH LOCAL ANESTHETIC DRUGS

Gilberto González Ramírez, MD[1,*] and Jaime Ruiz-Tovar, MD, PhD[2]

[1]Department of Bariatric Surgery Hospital Angeles del Carmen, Universidad de Guadalajara, Guadalajara, Mexico

[2]Department of Surgery, Universidad Autónoma de Madrid, Spain

ABSTRACT

Obesity surgery is and has been a challenge in all senses, since the conditions and the environment of the obese patient present their own and added difficulties due to the number of associated comorbidities. Therefore, the management of this type of patients must be multi-disciplinary at all times, always seeking to safeguard, improve and, in certain cases, cure patients of their condition. The above goes hand in hand with the processes that involve pre, intra and postoperative management in principle and then the relevant controls as well as the continuous monitoring. In this particular case we will discuss postoperative pain related to laparoscopic ports for adequate minimally invasive surgery, although the mere fact of being minimally invasive will

* Corresponding Author: Gilberto Gonzalez Ramirez, MD, Email: gilpchmd@yahoo.com.mx.

consequently result in less opening space and consequently pain, however multiple groups have been given the task of seeking to reduce postoperative pain related to laparoscopic ports, which has led to different techniques and times for the infiltration of local anesthetics in these ports, which by their own characteristics are the best analgesics both alone as in conjunction with other types of routes and medications to achieve adequate control and the patient can return to their activities and functionality necessary for a better postoperative course, which will generate better adaptation and therefore a positive evolution as well as a shorter hospital stay.

Although bariatric surgery is actually mainly performed laparoscopically, analgesic optimization continues being essential to reduce complications and to improve the patients' comfort. However, the adequate management of postoperative pain remains a major challenge, as it might condition the appearance of major morbidity, mainly pulmonary complications, leading to a decrease in the health-related quality of life in the immediate postsurgical period After every laparoscopic approach, there is a maximal peak of pain in the first 24 h after surgery, diminishing progressively after the 2nd–3rd postoperative days

Effective pain control encourages early ambulation, reducing the risk of thrombosis, and decreases pulmonary complications, such as atelectasia or pneumonia

The ease and safety of local anesthetics is well recognized and represent one of the most important classes of drug in perioperative care. Local anesthetic agents do not have the adverse effects of systemically administered opioids and act directly on the tissue to which they are applied.

Keywords: local anesthetics, infiltration, port sites, bariatric surgery

Introduction

Surgery for morbid obesity presents both surgeon and anesthesiologist a technical challenge. Physiologic responses to laparoscopic surgery, pneumoperitoneum, surgical complications, postoperative pain, and medical complications are some of the perioperative factors that affect recovery after bariatric surgery [1-3].

Although pain after laparoscopic surgery is less severe and of shorter duration than that after open surgery, it still causes considerable discomfort and increased stress response. The etiology of post laparoscopic pain can be classified into at least three aspects: visceral, incisional, and shoulder pain related to pneumoperitoneum [4-7]. The parietal pain is associated with the lesion in the abdominal wall during the insertion of the ports, visceral pain is related to the handling of the gastrointestinal serosa and the pain associated with the pneumoperitoneum causes a diaphragmatic irritation (by fluid, blood, or by the carbonic acid created from the mixing of carbon dioxide gas and intraperitoneal water) and stretching of the phrenic nerves during the procedure [8, 9]. It is usually located under the left shoulder.

It has been estimated that after laparoscopic surgery, parietal pain represents 50 – 70% of the total pain, visceral pain (10 – 20%) and the pain related to the pneumoperitoneum 20 – 30% [10-12].

Although visceral pain may also depend on the extent of intraabdominal surgery, incisional pain is related to the number and size of access devices and also to the technique of incision closure and drainage [4].

Minimizing Access-Related Pain

Pain from trocar placement is expected, but can be minimized by using the least number of ports required to perform the procedure safely, minimizing the number of large ports (i.e., ≥ 10 mm), and injecting local anesthetic at the port sites either before or at the end of the procedure [8, 13].

Port Design

Initially pyramidal cutting trocars were the mainstay. Trocars with shielded blades were then developed and are still the preferred port type in many centers. More recently, non- bladed trocars are increasingly being used as a growing number of studies suggest reduced complication rates.

These ports spread muscle and fascia rather than incise it and theoretically allow spontaneous re-approximation after trocar removal. A randomized prospective multicenter trial comparing radially expanding trocars to standard cutting trocars, in gastrointestinal surgery, has shown significantly reduced wound complications in the radial expansion group [14-16].

INNERVATION OF THE ABDOMINAL WALL: ANATOMICAL BACKGROUND

Laparoscopic techniques have revolutionized the field of surgery with benefits that include decreased postoperative pain, earlier return to normal activities following surgery, and fewer postoperative complications (i.e., wound infection, hernia) compared with open techniques [8-17].

Instrument mobility may also be limited depending upon the depth of the subcutaneous fat. Care must be taken during trocar placement to align them as needed for the procedure. Occasional repositioning of trocars may be necessary if procedures involve multiple abdominal quadrants [8]. More ports imply more pain.

The parietal peritoneum injury at the port sites may be a source of pain. For this reason, infiltration to around this level is preferable [18]. The walls of the abdomen are innervated by the last 6 intercostal nerves and the first lumbar nerve, they are mixed nerves and innerve parietal peritoneum, peripheral part of the diaphragmatic peritoneum and superficial planes on the part of the perforating branches [19].

The area of skin innervated by a spinal nerve is called a dermatome. Superimposition of contiguous dermatomes is observed, so that each segmental nerve is superimposed on the territory of its neighbor [19].

TOPIC INFILTRATION WITH LOCAL ANESTHETICS

In an effort to reduce the incidence and severity of postsurgical pain, multimodal analgesia has been defended by many authors, involving the use of two or more drugs with different mechanisms of action in an effort to maximize analgesic efficacy while reducing the risk and severity of adverse events [20]. These protocols include, among other measures, the association of intra- venous analgesia with epidural analgesia or the port sites infiltration with local anesthetic drugs [12, 21, 22].

Wound infiltration with local anesthetics proved to be a simple, effective, and inexpensive means of providing good analgesia in laparoscopic cholecystectomy, laparoscopic inguinal hernia repair, and gynecologic laparoscopic surgery. However, few studies have investigated its role in major laparoscopic surgery. To date, no study has investigated the benefits of wound infiltration in the setting of laparoscopic weight loss surgery [23-25].

In this chapter we will discuss only the infiltration of port site anesthetic drugs.

Choice of Local Anesthetics

The selection of an appropriate anesthetic will depend on several factors including: the time required for tissues adjacent to the area to be anesthetized, the mechanism of action and the routes of excretion of the drug to avoid complications. This is why it is important to know the necessary characteristics of each of the local anesthetics, for a correct and effective use when performing the different surgical procedures.

In this way, anesthetics are available for any of the requirements of the health professional. For example, in case of an infiltrative anesthesia, the use of lidocaine or bupivacaine is recommended [26-27].

Local anesthetics are drugs capable of reversibly blocking the conduction of the nerve impulse in any part of the nervous system to which they are applied, originating a temporary loss of sensitivity, which is recovered once finished the effect of the drug [27].

As for the pharmacokinetic properties of local anesthetics, their absorption depends both on the dose, as well as on the concentration and vascularization of the tissue where it is administered. Thus, the subcutaneous route is the one with the least absorption. Another of the elements that condition its absorption is the association with a vasoconstrictor drug [27].

Certain local anesthetics can be formulated in combination with epinephrine (adrenaline), a vasoconstrictor that reduces the systemic absorption of the drug. This combination is effective, especially in highly vascularized tissues, to reach higher concentrations of the drug in the administration site, prolong its anesthetic effect and, at the same time and reduce the adverse effects at the systemic level derived from its administration [27].

Local anesthetics of the amide group, such as ropivacaine, levobupicaine, bupivacaine, lidocaine, among others, are considered to last longer in their effect, unlike those of the ester group.

- Bupivacaine: It is a long-term local anesthetic indicated in subarachnoid anesthesia to perform interventions in the lower extremities, perineum and lower abdomen. It is also indicated in process anesthesia by infiltration or truncal block. Its main drawback is its potential cardiotoxicity.
- Levobupivacaine and ropivacaine: These are last generation local anesthetic drugs. They improve the safety profile (less cardiotoxicity and adverse effects at the central nervous system level). Ropivacaine is used in the treatment of acute pain and as an anesthetic agent in surgery (peripheral block, nerve trunk and epidural block); Levobupivacaine is used in local and regional anesthesia, as well as in numerous types of surgical and obstetric interventions. The efficacy of both drugs does not differ significantly from that of bupivacaine and their pharmacokinetic and pharmacodynamic profiles are also similar [27].

EFFECT OF PORT-SITE INFILTRATION WITH LOCAL ANESTHETIC DRUGS

Our group performed a previous study, involving patients undergoing a sleeve gastrectomy and compare the pain after the surgery with different analgesic approaches. All the interventions were performed laparoscopically [12].

In this study, the port sites infiltration was performed with 10 ml of bupivacaine 0.25%, applying 2 ml under the aponeurotic layer in each port. Patients were divided into three groups: Analgesia IV exclusively, epidural analgesia associated to analgesia IV and port- sites infiltration associated to analgesia IV (Group 3). A total of 147 patients were analyzed. There were no differences in age, gender, weight or BMI between groups. When analyzing the postoperative pain, patients presenting postoperative complications were excluded from the analysis, in order to reduce possible bias. Postoperative pain was assessed by Visual Analog Scale (VAS). Median pain 24 hours after surgery was 5 (range 3 – 8) in the patients receiving only analgesia IV, 2.5 (range 1 – 4) in those patients with epidural analgesia and 2 (range 0 – 4) in the group undergoing port sites infiltration with Bupivacaine associated to analgesia IV ($p = 0.01$). Pairwise analysis revealed that pain was significantly higher in the group receiving only analgesia IV, but there were no significant differences between epidural analgesia and port-site infiltration.

Referring to the morphine needs, in the group receiving only analgesia IV, it was necessary to administrate it in 16.3% patients, while in the other groups, it was necessary only in 2% ($P = 0.009$).

This study reflects that the patients receiving port sites infiltration with bupivacaine present an excellent pain relief, equivalent to that obtained in the patients with epidural analgesia. A correct pain control is essential to reduce surgical complications. Patients with adequate control relief can deambulate since the first postoperative day. The lack of morphine needs reduces postoperative nausea and vomits, allowing early oral intake.

Altogether, these facts may also possibly condition an earlier hospital discharge. The control of the postoperative pain is especially important in the morbidly obese patient, given that in these subjects the appearance of atelectasia and other lung complications is more frequent and might impair the sleep apnea/hypopnea syndrome [12, 28, 29].

Port sites infiltration with local anesthetics as analgesic method has also been described for many other laparoscopic procedures, as it is considered an easy, safe and cheap method. Notwithstanding, in these procedures, there is some controversy about its analgesic efficacy, existing series describing an excellent postoperative analgesia, but other authors could not demonstrate this efficacy [30-32].

Another controversial issue about port sites infiltration with local anesthetics is the optimal moment to apply the drug: at the beginning of the surgery, before performing the skin incisions, or when finishing the operation, before the skin suture [12]. The supporters of preincisional infiltration defend that the analgesic effect begins before performing the skin incisions, reducing the local inflammatory response secondary to the aggression caused by the skin incision and the introduction of the laparoscopic ports through the abdominal wall [33]. The anti-inflammatory effect of local anesthetics is not exactly known yet, but it has been hypothesized that it is mediated by the interaction of these drugs with cell membrane lipids and proteins, inducing an alteration of migration and adhesion of inflammatory cells to the vascular wall, and a reduction in the release of chemotactic agents, such as IL-6 or TNF-a, producing altogether a modulation in the systemic inflammatory response [34-35]. Sarac et al. [36] suggested that preemptive injection is not as effective as postoperative injection. However, recent reports support preemptive local infiltration. In a recent review article, it was affirmed that regarding pre- or postoperative wound injection, one is not more effective than the other [37-39].

Though bupivacaine is one of the local anesthetic drugs with longer duration, this usually does not prolong over 8 h after its administration, beginning the effect 5 – 10 min after the infiltration [40]. Therefore, if the operation time ranges between 60 and 180 min, the preincisional infiltration conditions a shorter analgesic effect postoperatively. This would explain why Moncada et al. [1] observed an analgesic effect only during the first 4 h after surgery, because part of the analgesic effect of the infiltration acted during the intervention, when it is unnecessary, because the patient is receiving other analgesic drugs. Moreover, the duration of the effect is also determined by the vascularization of the tissue where it is applied; the more vascularized the tissue, the drug passes earlier into the bloodstream and will be earlier metabolized in the liver and excreted by urine. The subaponeurotic space has few vascularization, similarly to the adipose tissue of the abdominal wall. When administrating the drug in the subaponeurotic space, it takes longer to disseminate and metabolize, possibly prolonging the analgesic effect beyond the 8 h expected. This preemptive or postoperative infiltration still remains a debatable issue [12].

Conclusion

Port sites infiltration with local anesthetics offers a means of postoperative analgesia that is practically harmless, easily reproducible, and can well be standardized. The infiltration at the beginning of surgery and at the end of it, is probably the best option. Preemptive infiltration might immunomodulate the release of inflammatory cytokines associated to the surgical damage, and postoperative one provides a long postoperative analgesia once finished the effect of the intraoperative drugs. Some local anesthetics combined with vasoconstrictors, such as adrenaline, might enhance its anesthetic effect and duration.

Current evidence suggests that this strategy should be employed in bariatric patient population as part of a multimodal postoperative pain management.

References

[1] Moncada, R; Martinaitis, L; Landecho, M; et al. Does Preincisional Infiltration with Bupivacaine Reduce Postoperative Pain in Laparoscopic Bariatric Surgery? *Obes Surg*, 2016, 26, 282-288.

[2] Schumann, R. Anaesthesia for bariatric surgery. *Best Pract Res Clin Anaesthesiol.* 2011, 25, 83–93.

[3] Levi, D; Goodman, ER; Patel, M; et al. Critical care of the obese and bariatric surgical patient. *Crit Care Clin.*, 2003, 19, 11–32.

[4] Neudecker, J; Sauerland, S. The European Association for Endoscopic Surgery clinical practice guideline on the pneumoperitoneum for laparoscopic surgery. *Surg Endosc*, 2002, 16, 1121-1143.

[5] Bisgaard, T; Klarskov, B; Kristiansen, VB; et al. Multi-regional local anesthetic infiltration during laparoscopic cholecystectomy in patients receiving prophylactic multi-modal analgesia: a randomized, double- blinded, placebo-controlled study. *Anesth Analg*, 1999, 89, 1017-1024.

[6] Joris, J; Thiry, E; Paris, P; et al. Pain after laparoscopic cholecystectomy: characteristics and effect of intra- peritoneal bupivacaine. *Anesth Analg*, 1995, 81, 379-384.

[7] Ure, BM; Troidl, H; Spangenberger, W; et al. Pain after laparoscopic cholecystectomy. Intensity and localization of pain and analysis of predictors in preoperative symptoms and intraoperative events. *Surg Endosc*, 1994, 8, 90-96.

[8] Telem, DA; Talamini, M; Gesten, F; et al. Hospital admissions greater than 30 days following bariatric surgery: patient and procedure matter. *Surg Endosc*, 2015, 29, 1310-1315.

[9] Jackson, SA; Laurence, AS; Hill, JC. Does post-laparoscopy pain relate to residual carbon dioxide? *Anaesthesia*, 1996, 51, 485-487.

[10] Joris, J; Thiry, E; Paris, P; et al. Pain after laparoscopic cholecystectomy: characteristics and effect of intraperitoneal bupivacaine. *Anesth Analg*, 1995, 81, 379–384.

[11] Mouton, WG; Bessel, JR; Otten, KT; et al. Pain after laparoscopy. *Surg Endosc*, 1999, 13, 445–448.

[12] Ruiz-Tovar, J; Muñoz, JL; Gonzalez, J; et al. Postoperative pain after laparoscopic sleeve gastrectomy: comparison of three analgesic schemes (isolated intravenous analgesia, epidural analgesia associated with intravenous analgesia and port-sites infiltration with

bupivacaine associated with intravenous analgesia) *Surg Endosc*, 2017, 31, 231–236.

[13] Neudecker, J; Sauerland, S; Neugebauer, E; et al. The European Association for Endoscopic Surgery clinical practice guideline on the pneumoperitoneum for laparoscopic surgery. *Surg Endosc*, 2002, 16, 1121-1143.

[14] Ibrahim, HM. Difficulties in Laparoscopic Access. In: Al-Kandari AM, Gill IS. *Difficult conditions in laparoscopic urologic surgery*, London, Springer-Verlag, 2011.

[15] Shafer, DM; Khajanchee, Y; Wong, J; Swanström, LL. Comparison of five different abdominal access trocar systems: analysis of insertion force, removal force and defect size. *Surg Innov.*, 2006, 13, 183-189.

[16] Leibl, BJ; Schmedt, CG; Schwarz, J; et al. Laparoscopic surgery complications associated with trocar tip design: review of literature and own results. *J Laparoendosc Adv Surg Tech A.*, 1999, 9, 135-140.

[17] Shabanzadeh, DM; Sørensen, LT. Laparoscopic surgery compared with open surgery decreases surgical site infection in obese patients: a systematic review and meta-analysis. *Ann Surg*, 2012, 256, 934-945.

[18] Alexander, DJ; Ngoi, SS; Lee, L; et al. Randomized trial of periportal peritoneal bupivacaine for pain relief after laparoscopic cholecystectomy. *Br J Surg.*, 1996, 83, 1223-1225.

[19] Koch, E; Jimenez, JC. Anatomía quirúrgica de las paredes anterolaterales del abdomen. *Buenos Aires, SACD*, 2009, 1-28.

[20] Practice guidelines for acute pain management in the postoperative setting: an updated report by the American Society of Anesthesiologists Task Force on acute pain management. *Anesthesiology*, 2012, 116, 248–273.

[21] Schumann, R; Shikora, S; Weiss, JM; et al. A comparison of multimodal perioperative analgesia to epidural pain management after gastric bypass surgery. *Anesth Analg*, 2003, 96, 469–474.

[22] Cantore, F; Boni, L; Di Giuseppe, M; et al. Pre-incisional local infiltration with levobupivacaine reduces pain and analgesic consumption after laparoscopic cholecystectomy: a new device for day-case procedure. *Int J Surg*, 2008, 6, 89–92.

[23] Gupta, A. Local anesthesia for pain relief after laparoscopic cholecystectomy—a systematic review. *Best Pract Res Clin Anaesthesiol.*, 2005, 19, 275–292.

[24] El Hachem, L; Small, E; Chung, P; et al. Randomized controlled double-blind trial of transversus abdominis plane block versus trocar site infiltration in gynecologic laparoscopy. *Am J Obstet Gynecol.*, 2015, 212, 182.e1-9.

[25] Cottam, DR; Fisher, B; Atkinson, J; et al. A randomized trial of bupivicaine pain pumps to eliminate the need for patient controlled analgesia pumps in primary laparoscopic Roux-en-Y gastric by-pass. *Obes Surg.*, 2007, 17, 595–600.

[26] Velásquez, P; Moreno, A. *Farmacología Básica y Clínica. Fármacos anestésicos locales.* Madrid, Editorial Médica Panamericana, 2005, 181 – 191. [*Basic and Clinical Pharmacology. Local anesthetic drugs.*]

[27] Katzung, G. Farmacología básica y clínica. Anestésicos Locales. México DF, Editorial El Manual Moderno S. A, 2007, 425-435. [*Basic and clinical pharmacology. Local anesthetics.*]

[28] Charghi, R; Backman, S; Christou, N; et al. Patient controlled iv analgesia is an acceptable pain management strategy in morbidly obese patients undergoing gastric bypass surgery. A retrospective comparison with epidural analgesia. *Can J Anesth*, 2003, 52, 672–678.

[29] Kehlet, H. The surgical stress response: should it be prevented? *Can J Surg*, 1991, 34, 565–567.

[30] Lee, IO; Kim, SH; Kong, MH; et al. Pain after laparoscopic cholecystectomy: the effect and timing of incisional and intraperitoneal bupivacaine. *Can J Anesth*, 2001, 48, 545–550.

[31] Jimenez Fuertes, M; Costa Navarro, D. Colecistectomıa laparoscopica ambulatoria y control del dolor postoperatorio:

presentacion de una serie de 100 casos. *Cir Esp*, 2015, 93, 181–186. [Ambulatory laparoscopic cholecystectomy and postoperative pain control: presentation of a series of 100 cases.]

[32] Tam, T; Harkins, G; Wegrzyniak, L; et al. Infiltration of bupivacaine local anesthetic to trocar insertion sites after laparoscopy: a randomized, double-blind, stratified, and controlled trial. *J Minim Invasive Gynecol*, 2014, 21, 1015–1021.

[33] Barczynsky, M; Konturek, A; Herman, RM. Superiority of preemptive analgesia with intraperitoneal instillation of bupivacaine before rather than after the creation of pneumoperitoneum for laparoscopic cholecystectomy: a randomized, double- blind, placebo-controlled study. *Surg Endosc*, 2006, 20, 1088–1093.

[34] Cassuto, J; Sinclair, R; Bonderovic, M. Anti-inflammatory properties of local anesthetics and their present a potential clinical implications. *Acta Anaesthesiol Scand*, 2006, 50, 265–282.

[35] Brocco, MC; Paulo, DN; Almeida, CE; et al. A study of interleukin 6 (IL-6) and tumor necrosis factor alpha (TNF-a) serum levels in rats subjected to fecal peritonitis and treated with intraperitoneal ropivacaine. *Acta Cir Bras*, 2012, 27, 494–498.

[36] Sarac, AM; Aktan, AO; Baykan, N; Yegen, C; Yalin, R. The effect and timing of local anesthesia in laparoscopic cholecystectomy. *Surg Laparosc Endosc*, 1996, 6, 362-366.

[37] Kato, J; Ogawa, S; Katz, H; et al. Effects of presurgical local infiltration of bupivacaine in the surgical field on postsurgical wound pain in laparoscopic gynecologic examinations: a possible preemptive analgesic effect. *Clin J Pain.*, 2000, 16, 12-17.

[38] Lee, IO; Kim, SH; Kong, MH; et al. Pain after laparoscopic cholecystectomy: the effect and timing of incisional and intraperitoneal bupivacaine. *Can J Anaesth.*, 2001, 48, 545-550.

[39] Wills, VL; Hunt, DR. Pain after laparoscopic cholecystectomy. *Br J Surg.*, 2000, 87, 273-284.

[40] Hodgson, PS; Liu, SS. New developments in spinal anesthesia. *Anesth Clin North Am*, 2000, 18, 235–249.

In: Management of Postoperative Pain … ISBN: 978-1-53614-284-6
Editor: Jaime Ruiz-Tovar

Chapter 7

LAPAROSCOPIC-GUIDED TRANSVERSUS ABDOMINIS PLANE (TAP) BLOCK AS PART OF MULTIMODAL ANALGESIA

***Jaime Ruiz-Tovar**, MD, PhD and Carolina Llavero*[2]**
[1]Department of Surgery, Universidad Autonoma de Madrid, Spain
[2]Department of Surgical Nursery, Garcilaso Clinic, Madrid, Spain

ABSTRACT

Transversus abdominis plane (TAP) blocks are an effective tool for the postoperative management of abdominal surgery, as they allow to block the sensitive nerves of the abdominal wall. These procedures are usually ultrasonographically-guided. However, in obese patients, the visualization of the abdominal wall muscles can be hindered and could lead to failed regional anesthesia. The laparoscopic-guided TAP has arisen as a method, allowing greater precision of needle placement in the desired tissue plane, obtaining an effective analgesia.

Keywords: transversus abdominis plane block, laparoscopic-guidance, postoperative pain

---

* Corresponding author: Jaime Ruiz-Tovar, MD, PhD. Email: jruiztovar@gmail.com.

INTRODUCTION

Bariatric surgery has been shown to be effective in achieving and maintaining weight loss and reducing obesity-related comorbidities [1, 2]. Bariatric surgery is mostly performed laparoscopically. It has been demonstrated that the laparoscopic approach is associated with lower complication rates, shorter hospital stays and earlier reincorporation to normal activities than after open procedures [3]. However, the adequate management of postoperative pain remains a major challenge, as it might condition the appearance of major morbidity, mainly pulmonary complications, leading to a decrease in the health-related quality of life in the immediate postsurgical period [4].

Therefore, in an effort to reduce the incidence and severity of postsurgical pain, multimodal analgesia, as part of Enhanced Recovery After Surgery (ERAS) programs, has been defended by many authors. Multimodal analgesia involves the use of two or more drugs with different mechanisms of action in an effort to maximize analgesic efficacy while reducing the risk and severity of adverse events [5, 6]. These protocols applied to laparoscopic bariatric surgery mostly include the association of intravenous analgesia with the port-sites infiltration with local anesthetic drugs [7]. A previous study of our group demonstrated that port-site infiltration with bupivacaine associated with intravenous analgesia achieves a significantly better pain control than intravenous analgesia alone [8].

The transversus abdominis plane (TAP) block is a regional anesthetic technique that targets the sensory nerve supply of the anterior-lateral abdominal wall. The block is performed by injecting local anesthetic into the plane between the internal oblique and the transversus abdominis muscles using the triangle of Petit as a landmark. This TAP plane is infiltrated with local anesthetics to target the T7–T12 intercostal nerves, the ilioinguinal, iliohypogastric, and the lateral cutaneous branches of the dorsal rami of L1–L3 [9, 10].

TAP blocks have been successfully implemented for pain control after laparoscopic surgery in non-obese patients undergoing diverse procedures

[11]. The resulting analgesia may be especially beneficial in morbidly obese patients after abdominal surgery due to their higher risk for postoperative pulmonary complication [12, 13]. The introduction of ultrasound guidance has allowed greater precision of needle placement in the desired tissue plane [14]. However, visualization of the abdominal wall muscles can be hindered by morbid obesity and could lead to failed regional anesthesia [15].

Recently, we undertook a study to determine the feasibility of using laparoscopic-guided TAP blocks in patients with morbid obesity undergoing Roux-en-Y gastric bypass (RYGB) and compare its analgesic effect postoperatively with the classical method of port-site infiltration. A prospective randomized clinical trial of patients undergoing RYGB at a single institution, was performed. Patients undergoing other bariatric techniques, with previous foregut surgery and patients presenting postoperative complications were excluded. Patients were randomized into 2 groups: those patients undergoing laparoscopic-guided TAP associated to intravenous analgesia (TAP lap Group) and those ones receiving intravenous analgesia associated with port-sites infiltration (PSI Group).

SURGICAL TECHNIQUE

5 ports will be placed in right hypochondrium (12 mm), left hypochondrium (12 mm), epigastrium (11 mm), subxyphoideal (11 mm), and left flank (5 mm). Pneumoperitoneum pressure was established in 12 mmHg. A 6-cm long gastric pouch was performed, calibrating it with a 36-Fr bougie, with a linear stapler (Echelon Flex, Johnson & Johnson, USA). A 60-cm biliary limb and a 150-cm alimentary limb were performed. Both anastomoses were performed with linear stapler (Echelon Flex, Johnson & Johnson, USA), calibrating the gastrojejunal anastomosis at 2 cm. Mesenteric defects were not closed in any of the cases. The integrity of the anastomoses and staple lines were checked with intraoperative methylene blue dye; postoperative tests were not used.

Analgesic Technique

Intravenous analgesia included Metamizole 2g/8h and Acetaminophen 1g/8h, alternating every 4 hours.

Port-sites infiltration was performed with 30 ml of Bupivacaine 0.25%, applying 6 ml under the aponeurotic layer in each port.

TAP lap was performed with 30 ml of Bupivacaine 0.25%, applying it into the plane between the internal oblique and the transversus abdominis muscles. The injection was performed at 3 levels, coinciding with the same dermatomes where the port-sites were located. The injection was performed at the dermatomes, but lateral to the port-sites. The infiltration was performed bilaterally with a volume of 5ml in each injection place. The laparoscopic guidance consists in the insertion of the needle until the tip protrudes on the peritoneal layer, without traversing it. Then the needle is retracted 3mm into the abdominal wall, which is the estimated thickness of the preperitoneal space and the transversus abdominis muscle, so that the anesthetic is injected into the space between the internal oblique muscle and the transversus abdominis muscle. The injection of the anesthetic drug into this space induces the formation of a bulge, observed as a mild protrusion in the abdominal wall towards the peritoneum. The mild protrusion indicates that the injection place is correct, as shown in the following figures. A greater protrusion indicates that the drug has been injected in the preperitoneal space. In order to validate the technique, in the first 10 patients the injections in the correct spaces were confirmed with ultrasonography.

When postoperative pain, as measured by VAS, overcame 50 mm at any moment in the postoperative course, 5mg of subcutaneous morphine was administrated.

Analyzed variables in the study included age, gender, anthropometric values (weight, BMI), operation time, postoperative complications, mortality, hospital stay, pain quantification as measured by Visual Analogic Scale (VAS), ranging from 0 (absence of pain) to 10 (unbearable pain) 24 hours after surgery, and morphine needs during the first 24 hours.

Pain quantification during the first 24 hours was evaluated by a nurse blinded to the treatment applied.

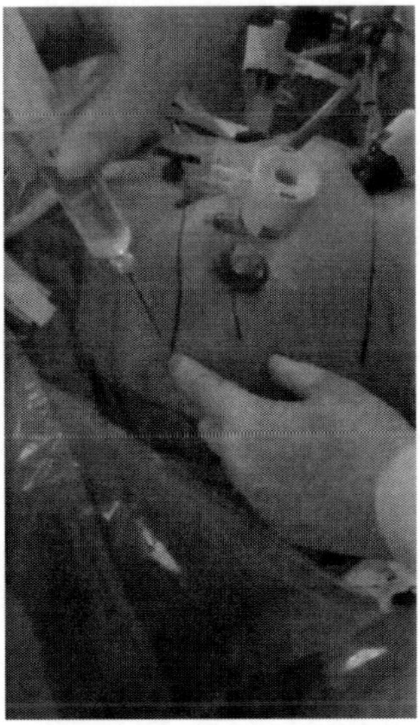

Figure 1. The injection is performed at 3 levels, coinciding with the same dermatomes where the port-sites were located, and lateral to them. The infiltration was performed bilaterally.

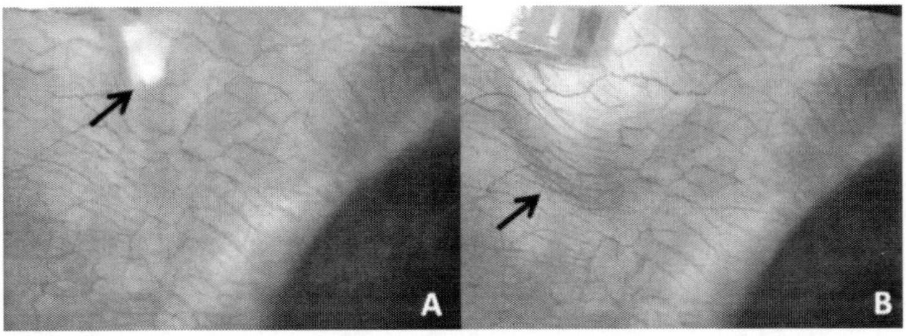

Figure 2. A: The laparoscopic guidance consists in the insertion of the needle until the tip protrudes on the peritoneal layer, without traversing it. B: Then the needle is retracted 3mm into the abdominal wall, which is the estimated thickness of the preperitoneal space and the transversus abdominis muscle, so that the anesthetic is injected into the space between the internal oblique muscle and the transversus abdominis muscle. The injection of the anesthetic drug into this space induces the formation of a bulge, observed as a mild protrusion in the abdominal wall towards the peritoneum.

A total of 140 patients were included, 70 in each group, consisting in 80 females (57.1%) and 60 males (42.9%), with a mean age of 41.8 $\pm$ 7.3 years and a mean BMI of 47 $\pm$ 4.5 Kg/m^2. There were no differences in age, gender, comorbidities, weight or BMI between groups.

Mean operative time was 83.3 $\pm$ 15.6 min in TAP lap and 80.5 $\pm$ 14.4 min in PSI (NS). Mean postoperative pain, as measured by VAS, 24 hours after surgery was 16.8 $\pm$ 11.2mm in PSI and 10 $\pm$ 8.1mm in TAP-lap ($p = 0.001$). Morphine rescues were necessary in 13.2% in PSI and 2.9% in TAP-lap (OR 4.96; CI95% (2.3 – 11.2); $p = 0.026$). Mean hospital stay was 2.1 $\pm$ 1.2 days in TAP-lap and 2.9 $\pm$ 1.3 days in PSI ($p = 0.019$). Hospital discharge during the first 48h after surgery was possible in 52.9% of the patients in PSI and 71% in TAP-lap (OR 4.75; CI95% (2.1 - 10.8); $p = 0.029$).

Postoperative pain after bariatric surgery presents 3 components: parietal pain associated to the lesion in the abdominal wall during the insertion of the ports, visceral pain related with the handling of the gastrointestinal serosa, and the pain associated to the pneumoperitoneum, causing a diaphragmatic irritation and usually located under the left shoulder. It has been estimated that after laparoscopic surgery, parietal pain represents 50 - 70% of the total pain, visceral pain (10 - 20%) and the pain related to the pneumoperitoneum 20 - 30% [16, 17].

Port-sites infiltration with local anesthetics as analgesic method, has been described for many laparoscopic procedures as a method to reduce the parietal pain. It is considered an easy, safe and cheap method. Notwithstanding, there is some controversy about its analgesic efficacy, existing series describing an excellent postoperative analgesia [18, 19], but other authors could not demonstrate this efficacy [20]. Specifically referring to bariatric surgery, a publication of a Spanish group reports that the association of port-sites infiltration with bupivacaine achieves a reduction of postoperative pain during the first 4 hours, but they did not observe differences after this time. Systemic absorption and peak plasma levels of local anesthetic following blocks in bariatric patients have not been analyzed, but this would not be probably associated with the efficacy and duration of the analgesia, as the effect is mainly local, with the direct contact of the drug with the nerve fiber, blocking nerve conduction by reducing the membrane permeability to sodium [21]. The main problem of port-site infiltration is that the subaponeurotic administration of the drug is performed in a blind manner, especially in morbidly obese patients, as the aponeurotic layer cannot be seen at the time of the infiltration and the aponeurosis placement is just estimated as a point of higher resistance during the introduction of the needle. To minimize this estimative infiltration, the ultrasonographic guidance has been developed in order to clearly visualize the placement of drug injection.

Andersen et al. [22] performed a recent systematic review of randomized trials involving the analgesic treatment in laparoscopic gastric bypass surgery. Though the methodological quality of most included studies was limited, they conclude that the administration of nonsteroidal anti-inflammatory drugs, local anesthetics (intraperitoneally or subfascially/subcutaneously), transversus abdominis plane block, dexmedetomidine, and ketamine may improve analgesia compared to placebo. No studies compared the different analgesic schemes between them, but many anesthesiologists defend TAP blockade as superior to port-site infiltration and, if they are going to perform an ultrasound-guided infiltration, they prefer to carry out a TAP block rather than a port site infiltration.

The TAP block has been previously studied in patients having different open and laparoscopic surgical procedures. Most studies have demonstrated that the TAP block decreases peri- and postoperative pain and reduces the use of opioids [11]. Recent studies have shown similar benefits in obese patients undergoing laparoscopic colorectal surgery and Cesarean delivery [23, 24]. Several authors defend that ultrasound guidance allow identification of the layers of the abdominal wall even in obese patients, where landmarks are often obscured by the body habitus [25]. However, due to deep anatomic location of structures and nerves, the ultrasound beam travels a greater distance, leading to beam attenuation. Moreover, the image quality through fat may be poorer as the adipose tissue has a nonlinear relationship to frequency, whereas most biological tissues have linear relationship. In addition, the irregularly shaped adipose layers leads to uneven speed of sound causing phase aberration of the sound field. So that above the focus of the transducer, there is differing speeds of sound, leading to mismatch of acoustic impedance at the fat/muscle interfaces. In obese patients, there is an increase in the number of reflective interfaces not only leading to more echoes but also decreasing the incident of sound available to penetrate deeper tissues, such as nerves, vessels, or other targeted structures [26-28]. In our experience, many anesthesiologists refer difficulties in the identification of the transversus abdominis plane when performing ultrasound-guided TAP blocks, because of the great thickness of the subcutaneous adipose tissue. Thus, we decided to perform this procedure with laparoscopic guidance. It is true that laparoscopic guidance is not as exact as ultrasound one, as the muscular layers cannot be identified. We just identify the tip of the needle when protruding on the peritoneum and we retract it 3mm, based on the estimated thickness of the transversus abdominis muscle and the preperitoneal space. Moreover, the bulge obtained must suggest that the infiltration is not performed in the preperitoneal layer, that will provoke a greater bulge, nor in the space between both oblique muscles, that will not perform any bulge as the internal oblique muscle has greater thickness that the transversus abdominis. To validate our technique, the correct injection place was confirmed with ultrasonography.

Said et al. have recently published a novel method of continuous TAP blocks via laparoscopically-placed catheters for bariatric surgery. They performed a laparoscopic dissection of the space between transversus abdominis and internal oblique muscles, placing there a catheter for continuous infusion of local anesthetics, and obtained a significant reduction of postoperative pain and opioid needs. In the performance of this approach, these authors confirm that the transverses abdominis muscle has a width of 2-3mm, as we hypothesized in our technique and the infusion tests they performed with normal saline, obtained similar bulging images than in our patients [29].

Laparoscopic-guided TAP block implied in our patients a lower postoperative pain and lower requirements of opioid rescues, consequently leading to a shorter hospital stay and a hospital discharge within the first 48 hours after the surgery in 71% of the patients. These results suggest that laparoscopic-guided TAP block is a useful tool for the multimodal management of postoperative pain. The main limitation of the technique is that it is operator-dependent and requires a certain learning curve or validation in the first cases with ultrasonography, in order to confirm the infiltration in the correct space.

CONCLUSION

Laparoscopic-guided TAP block reduces postoperative pain, opioid needs and hospital stays when compared with port-site infiltration with the same anesthetic drug, without increasing operation time. It can be considered a useful tool in the multimodal management of postoperative pain after bariatric surgery.

REFERENCES

[1] Bray, GA. Medical consequences of obesity. *J Clin Endocrinol Metab*, 2004, 89, 2583–2589.

[2] Sullivan, PW; Ghushchyan, VH; Ben-Joseph, R. The impact of obesity on diabetes, hyperlipidemia and hypertension in the United States. *Qual Life Res*, *17*, 1063–1071.

[3] Cantore, F; Boni, L; Di Giuseppe, M; et al. Pre-incisional local infirltration with levobupivacaine reduces pain and analgesic consumption after laparoscopic cholecystectomy: a new device for day-case procedure. *Int J Surg*, 2008, 6, 89–92.

[4] Bertin, PM. Liposome bupivacaine for postsurgical pain in an obese woman with chronic pain undergoing laparoscopic gastrectomy: a case report. *J Med Case Rep*, 2014, 8, 21–25.

[5] Wu, CL; Naqibuddin, M; Rowlingson, AJ; et al. The effect of pain on health-related quality of life in immediate postoperative period. *Anesth Analg*, 2003, 97, 1078–1085.

[6] Practice guidelines for acute pain management in the postoperative setting: an updated report by the American Society of Anesthesiologists Task Force on acute pain management. *Anesthesiology*, 2012, 116, 248–273.

[7] Schumann, R; Shikora, S; Weiss, JM; et al. A comparison of multimodal perioperative analgesia to epidural pain management after gastric bypass surgery. *Anesth Analg*, 2003, 96, 469–474.

[8] Ruiz-Tovar, J; Muñoz, JL; Gonzalez, J; et al. Postoperative pain after laparoscopic sleeve gastrectomy: comparison of three analgesic schemes (isolated intravenous analgesia, epidural analgesia associated with intravenous analgesia and port-sites infiltration with bupivacaine associated with intravenous analgesia). *Surg Endosc*, 2017, 31, 231-236.

[9] McDonnell, JG; O'Donnell, BD; Farrell, T; et al. Transversus abdominis plane block: a cadaveric and radiological evaluation. *Reg Anesth Pain Med.*, 2007, 32, 399–404.

[10] El-Dawlatly, AA; Turkistani, A; Kettner, SC; et al. Ultrasound-guided transversus abdominis plane block: description of a new technique and comparison with conventional systemic analgesia during laparoscopic cholecystectomy. *Br J Anaesth.*, 2009, 102, 763–767.

[11] Wassef, M; Lee, DY; Levine, JL; et al. Feasibility and analgesic efficacy of the transversus abdominis plane block after single-port laparoscopy in patients having bariatric surgery. *J Pain Res*, 2013, 6, 837–841.

[12] Ahmad, S; Nagle, A; McCarthy, RJ; et al. Postoperative hypoxemia in morbidly obese patients with and without obstructive sleep apnea undergoing laparoscopic bariatric surgery. *Anesth Analg.*, 2008, 107, 138–143.

[13] Rosenberg-Adamsen, S; Lie, C; Bernhard, A; et al. Effect of oxygen treatment on heart rate after abdominal surgery. *Anaesthesiology.*, 1999, 90, 380–384.

[14] Hadzic, A. *Textbook of Regional Anesthesia and Acute Pain Management.* 1st ed. New York: McGraw-Hill, 2007.

[15] Nielsen, KC; Guller, U; Steele, SM; et al. Influence of obesity on surgical regional anesthesia in the ambulatory setting: an analysis of 9,038 blocks. *Anaesthesiology.*, 2005, 102, 181–187.

[16] Joris, J; Thiry, E; Paris, P; et al. Pain after laparoscopic cholecystectomy: characteristics and effect of intraperitoneal bupivacaine. *Anesth Analg*, 1995, 81, 379-384.

[17] Mouton, WG; Bessel, JR; Otten, KT; et al. Pain after laparoscopy. *Surg Endosc*, 1999, 13, 445-448.

[18] Lee, IO; Kim, SH; Kong, MH; et al. Pain after laparoscopic cholecystectomy: the effect and timing of incisional and intraperitoneal bupivacaine. *Can J Anesth*, 2001, 48, 545-550.

[19] Jimenez Fuertes, M; Costa Navarro, D. Colecistectomía laparoscópica ambulatoria y control del dolor postoperatorio: presentación de una serie de 100 casos. *Cir Esp*, 2015, 93, 181-186. [Ambulatory laparoscopic cholecystectomy and postoperative pain control: presentation of a series of 100 cases]

[20] Tam, T; Harkins, G; Wegrzyniak, L; et al. Infiltration of bupivacaine local anesthetic to trocar insertion sites after laparoscopy: a randomized, double-blind, stratified, and controlled trial. *J Minim Invasive Gynecol*, 2014, 21, 1015-1021.

[21] Moncada, R; Martinaitis, L; Landecho, M; et al. Does preincisional infiltration with bupivacaine reduce postoperative pain in laparoscopic bariatric surgery? *Obes Surg*, 2016, 26, 282-288.

[22] Andersen, LP; Werner, MU; Rosenberg, J; et al. Analgesic treatment in laparoscopic gastric bypass surgery: a systematic review of randomized trials. *Obes Surg*, 2014, 24, 462-470.

[23] Singh, S; Dhir, S; Marmai, K; Rehou, S; Silva, M; Bradbury, C. Efficacy of ultrasound-guided transversus abdominis plane blocks for post-cesarean delivery analgesia: a double-blind, dose-comparison, placebo-controlled randomized trial. *Int J Obstet Anesth.*, 2013, 22, 188–193.

[24] Walter, CJ; Maxwell-Armstrong, C; Pinkney, TD; et al. A randomised controlled trial of the efficacy of ultrasound-guided

transversus abdominis plane (TAP) block in laparoscopic colorectal surgery. *Surg Endosc.*, 2013, 27, 2366–2372.

[25] Sinha, A; Jayaraman, L; Punhani, D. Efficacy of ultrasound-guided transversus abdominis plane block after laparoscopic bariatric surgery: a double blind, randomized, controlled study. *Obes Surg.*, 2013, 23, 548–553.

[26] Saranteas, T. Limitations in ultrasound imaging techniques in anesthesia: obesity and muscle atrophy? *Anesth Analg.*, 2009, 108, 660–5.

[27] Feigenbaum, H. Physics and instrumentation. In: Feingenbaum H, Armstrong WF, Rayan T, editors. *Feigenbaum's echocardiography*. Philadelphia: Lippincott William and Wilkins, 2005, p. 12–5.

[28] Shmulewitz, A; Teefey, SA; Robinson, BS. Factors affecting image quality and diagnostic efficacy in abdominal sonography: a prospective study of 140 patients. *J Clin Ultrasound.*, 1993, 21, 623–30.

[29] Said, AM; Balamoun, HA. Comntinuous trasnversus abdominis plane blocks via laparoscopically placed catheters for bariatric surgery. *Obes Surg*, 2017, 27, 2575-2582.

In: Management of Postoperative Pain ... ISBN: 978-1-53614-284-6
Editor: Jaime Ruiz-Tovar

Chapter 8

The Effect of Peritoneal Irrigation with Ropivacaine

Montiel Jiménez-Fuertes, MD, PhD
Department of Digestive Surgery,
Rey Juan Carlos University Hospital, Móstoles (Madrid), Spain

Abstract

Postoperative pain is a problem after laparoscopy, with direct consequences on the patient's quality of life and on health care cost. Intraperitoneal use of local anesthetic drugs has been associated with the reduction of postoperative pain, and the ropivacain has been related with reduction of pain and analgesic drugs comsumption after laparoscopic surgery.

Keywords: postoperative pain, ropivacaine, local anesthetics

Introduction

Postoperative pain is a problem after laparoscopy, with direct consequences on the patient's quality of life and on health care cost. Pain after laparoscopic surgery is usually attributed to surgical manipulations, including intraperitoneal insufflation of carbon dioxide, resulting in peritoneal stretching, diaphragmatic irritation, changes in intra-abdominal pH, and retention of the insufflated gas within the abdominal cavity after surgery, and also from the incision sites [1]. These manipulations also result in the irritation of peritoneal nerves causing visceral and shoulder pain. Previous studies have reported that as many as 80% of patients required opioid analgesia after laparoscopic surgery, which also may increase postoperative morbidity and hospital stay [2].

Several studies regarding the intraperitoneal instillation and intraperitoneal nebulization of ropivacaine during several laparoscopic procedures such as colectomy, appendectomy, cholecystectomy, bariatric surgery and gynecologic procedures, even laparoscopic procedures in children, has been associated with reduction of pain and analgesic consumption [3-12].

ROPIVACAINE

Ropivacaine is a long-acting regional anesthetic that is structurally related to Bupivacaine. It is a pure S(-)enantiomer, unlike Bupivacaine, which is a racemate, developed for the purpose of reducing potential toxicity and improving relative sensory and motor block profiles [13].

Mechanism of Action

Ropivacaine causes reversible inhibition of sodium ion influx, and thereby blocks impulse conduction in nerve fibers [14]. This action is potentiated by dose-dependent inhibition of potassium channels [15]. Ropivacaine is less lipophilic than bupivacaine and is less likely to penetrate large myelinated motor fibers; therefore, it has selective action on the pain-transmitting A β and C nerves rather than Aβ fibers, which are involved in motor function.

Pharmcodinamics

Central Nervous System (CNS) and Cardiovascular Effects

Ropivacaine is less lipophilic than bupivacaine and that, together with its stereoselective properties, contributes to ropivacaine having a significantly higher threshold for cardiotoxicity and CNS toxicity than bupivacaine in animals and healthy volunteers [16].

The lower lipophilicity of ropivacaine versus bupivacaine correlated with the lesser cardiodepressant effects of both ropivacaine isomers than of the bupivacaine isomers in animal studies [17].

The CNS effects occurred earlier than cardiotoxic symptoms during an intravenous (IV) infusion of local anesthetic (10 mg/min of ropivacaine or bupivacaine) in human volunteers and the infusion was stopped at this point. Significant changes in cardiac function involving the contractility, conduction time and QRS width occurred and the increase in a QRS width was found to be significantly smaller with ropivacaine than with bupivacaine [18, 19].

Other Effects

Ropivacaine has been shown to inhibit platelet aggregation in plasma at concentrations of 3.75 and 1.88 mg/mL (0.375% and 0.188%), which correspond to those that could occur in the epidural space during infusion [20]. Like other anesthetics, ropivacaine has antibacterial activity *in vitro*, inhibiting the growth of *Staphylococcus aureus*, [21, 22] *Escherichia coli* [21], and *Pseudomonas aeruginosa* [22].

Pharmacikinetics

Absorption and Distribution

The plasma concentration of ropivacaine depends on the total dose administered and the route of administration, as well as the hemodynamic and circulatory condition of the patient and vascularity of the administration site [23].

When ropivacaine was administered intravenously in subjects, its pharmacokinetics were linear and dose proportional up to 80 mg [23]. The absorption of ropivacaine 150 mg from the epidural space is complete and biphasic. The mean half-life of the initial phase is approximately 14 minutes, followed by a slower phase with a mean absorption $t_{1/2}$ of approximately 4.2 hours.

Ropivacaine is bound to plasma proteins to an extent of 94%, mainly to α1-acid glycoprotein. The total plasma concentration increase during continuous epidural infusion of ropivacaine [23, 24] is caused by an increase in the degree of protein binding and subsequent decrease in clearance of ropivacaine [24].

Ropivacaine rapidly crosses the placenta during epidural administration for caesarean section, resulting in near complete equilibrium of the free fraction of ropivacaine in the maternal and fetal circulation [25]. However, the total plasma concentration of ropivacaine was lower in the fetal circulation than in the maternal circulation, reflecting the binding of ropivacaine to α1-acid glycoprotein, which is more concentrated in maternal than in fetal plasma.

Regarding to the instillation and nebulization of ropivacaine, although the exact mechanism of action is not fully understood, it is probably through the effects of the local anesthetic on peritoneal nerve endings, which may involve local and systemic modulation of the inflammatory process.

Metabolism and Excretion

Ropivacaine is metabolized extensively in the liver, predominantly by aromatic hydroxylation to 3'-hydroxy-ropivacaine by cytochrome P450 (CYP) 1A2 and N-dealkylation to 2,'6'-pipecoloxylidide by CYP3A4 [16, 17]. The kidney is the main excretory organ for ropivacaine, accounting for 86% of the excretion of the drug in urine after a single intravenous dose administration. It has a mean ± SD terminal half-life of 1.8 ± 0.7 h and 4.2 ± 1.0 h after intravenous and epidural administration, respectively.

Relative Potency

A strict correlation exists between the lipid solubility of the local anesthetic and its potency and toxicity. According to minimum local anesthetic concentration (MLAC) studies, which are based on effective analgesia in 50% of patients) ropivacaine has similar potency to bupivacaine at higher doses (e.g., doses required for peripheral nerve blocks for surgical anesthesia), ropivacaine is less potent than bupivacaine and levobupivacaine at lower doses, such as those used for epidural or intrathecal analgesia. Providing anesthesia or analgesia for the majority of patients is more clinically relevant than the MLAC and, at higher doses used in clinical practice, this potency difference is not always evident.

INTRAPERITONEAL ROPIVACAIN INSTILLATION

Intraperitoneal local anesthetics are now widely used in several laparoscopic procedures, as they provide the benefit of analgesia without systemic side effects that may result from use of enterally and parenterally administered drugs [26].

Various local anesthetics such as lignocaine, bupivacaine, ropivacaine, and levobupivacaine have been evaluated in many trials. Several factors are important for intraperitoneal instillation of drug to decrease postoperative pain, which include choice of drug, concentration of drug, volume of drug, and timing of drug administration [27, 28].

Timing of intraperitoneal instillation of local anesthetic is very important. Barczynski et al. evaluated the optimal timing of bupivacaine peritoneal instillation and concluded that peritoneal instillation was much more effective for pain relief if used before creation of pneumoperitoneum [29]. Maestroni et al. also studied preemptive analgesia in LC where both local anesthetic and normal saline (NS) were administered before creation of pneumoperitoneum and suggested only application before creation of pneumoperitoneum may preempt every neuronal central sensitization [30]. The patients receiving intraperitoneal ropivacaine before creation of pnemoperitoneum had lesser pain in the first 12 h during the postoperative period [31, 32]. In this sense, preemptive analgesia with intraperitoneal instillation of ropivacaine in saline before the creation of pneumoperitoneum has improved surgical outcome after laparoscopic cholecystectomy in terms of significantly diminished total abdominal and shoulder tip pain, decreased analgesia request and analgesic consumption [31].

The use of ropivacaine for intraperitoneal instillation has been extended more than others because of its low toxicity and longer duration of action. Ropivacaine is a long-acting amide type local anesthetic used as regional anesthetic. It is a pure S(−) enantiomer, developed for the purpose of reducing potential cardiac toxicity and improving relative sensory and motor block profiles. When ropivacaine is given intraperitoneally it starts acting within 10–20 min, and duration of action lasts for 4–6 h. Kucuk et al. have found that intraperitoneal instillation of 150 mg of ropivacaine was significantly more effective than either 100 mg bupivacaine or 100 mg ropivacaine for preventing postoperative pain [33]. Another important aspect is the appropriate volume of the medium used for instillation. It should be large enough to reach the entire subdiaphragmatic region. Some studies have shown that better abdominal and shoulder tip pain control was observed when larger volume of local anesthetic solution was used for instillation rather than smaller volume [32].

In a recent meta-analysis, Young et al. [34] reported that the pain at 4-8 h and at 9-24 h were significantly reduced in the intraperitoneal ropivacaine instillation. Thus, it appears that intraperitoneal ropivacaine instillation may have a slight effect in promoting the Enhanced Recovery after Surgery (ERAS) since patients undergoing day-surgery laparoscopic cholecystectomy are discharged between four and 8 h after surgery. They found that the rate of adverse events in studies of ropivacaine intraperitoneal instillation are low and reduces pain in people undergoing laparoscopic cholecystectomy. A review by Kahokehr et al. concluded that intraperitoneal local anesthetic instillation reduced pain and no further trials were necessary [35]. Another review reported that intraperitoneal instillation of local anesthetic resulted in a reduction of the mean pain score [36].

Choi et al. [37] concluded in their meta-analysis that intraperitoneal local anesthetics in patients undergoing laparoscopic cholecystectomy exhibited beneficial effects on post-operative abdominal, visceral, and shoulder pain in a resting state. Ahn et al. [38] reported that preoperative use of intraperitoneal LA, e.g., at the time induction of anesthesia was better than its use at the end of procedure. Bucciero et al. [39] found that intraperitoneal ropivacaine nebulization was associated with reduced shoulder pain as compared to instillation group and unassisted walking after LC. So the evidence favors that at intraperitoneal location, LA should be used before creation of pneumoperitoneum and nebulization is better than instillation.

This is an emerging concept that the use of LA both at the incision site as well as intraperitoneally provides better pain relief. Hence, multiregional anesthesia seems desirable, and the use of drug at both sites seem to cater to different pain components and provide analgesia by two different mechanisms so their effect in pain relief may be additive [40].

Dosage of Ropivacaine for Peritoneal Instillation

Ropivacaine has been used in variable amounts and in variable concentrations by various authors [29-41]. There is no clear cut consensus on this, and intraperitoneal ropivacaine doses varied from 40 to 300 mg.

INTRAPERITONEAL ROPIVACAIN NEBULIZATION

Local anesthetic instillation can provide pain relief after laparoscopic surgery, but local anesthetic distribution may not always be uniform throughout the peritoneal surface [38]. Intraperitoneal local anesthetic nebulization is a relatively novel approach to pain management after laparoscopic surgery. This approach should provide uniform dispersion of local anesthetic particles throughout the peritoneal cavity [41-44]. However, the analgesic effectiveness of intraperitoneal local anesthetic nebulization may depend upon the nebulization device and the delivery mode. Alkhamesi and colleagues [44] reported that nebulization of bupivacaine using a custom-made device significantly reduced pain after laparoscopic cholecystectomy. Compared with intraperitoneal ropivacaine instillation, nebulization of ropivacaine using a high-frequency vibrating membrane nebulizer (Aeroneb Prow, Aerogen, Galway, Ireland) reduced shoulder pain and the time to unassisted walking after laparoscopic cholecystectomy [41-44]. In contrast, Zimmer and colleagues [45] did not find significant differences in pain or analgesic consumption after bupivacaine nebulization using the Insuflow device, which is a hot evaporation-based nebulizer. It is not surprising that these authors did not observe any analgesic benefits from nebulizing bupivacaine 0.5% (10 ml), because hot evaporation enables only evaporation of the solvent (e.g., water) and not of the solute (e.g., local anesthetic), thus making the device inefficient in delivering the local anesthetic into the peritoneal cavity. This suggests that studies evaluating the effects of peritoneal nebulization should use a device suitable to deliver the local anesthetic.

One of the limitations of the nebulization technique is that the small size of droplets creates a 'foggy' environment, which may interfere with the surgeon's vision [46]. Thus, continuous local anesthetic nebulization throughout the surgical duration is not clinically feasible. Therefore, we performed the initial nebulization through the central port during the insertion of the other ones, and the second nebulization just before exsufflation of the pneumoperitoneum.

Regarding to the dose, Ingelmo et al. [47] used 30 mg of ropivacaine based upon previous reports and upon the time taken by surgeons for port placement (Aeroneb Pro can deliver 3 ml of solution in 5–6 min). Although superior analgesia may be obtained by larger doses of local anesthetics, this would require a longer nebulization time, which may delay the start of surgery. Future studies should include a dose-finding analysis, the evaluation of the pharmacokinetics profile of different doses of ropivacaine, and the impact on the surgeon's vision of different nebulization times.

Conclusion

Intraperitoneal ropivacaine instillation and nebulization seem to reduce postoperative pain after laparoscopic surgery in several procedures.

References

[1] Kandaswamy, R. Laparoscopic vs open nephrectomy in 210 consecutive patients: outcomes, cost, and changes in practice patterns. *Surg Endosc*. 2004; 18(11):1684-8.

[2] Joris J, Cigarini I, Legrand M, Jacquet N, De Groote D, Franchimont P et al. Metabolic and respiratory changes after cholecystectomy performed via laparotomy or laparoscopy. *Br J Anaesth*. 1992; 69(4):341-5.

[3] Kahokehr A, Sammour T, Zargar Shoshtari K, Taylor M, Hill AG. Intraperitoneal local anesthetic improves recovery after colon resection: a double-blinded randomized controlled trial. *Ann Surg*. 2011;254(1):28-38.

[4] Kang H, Kim BG. Intraperitoneal ropivacaine for effective pain relief after laparoscopic appendectomy: a prospective, randomized, double-blind, placebo-controlled study. *J Int Med Res*. 2010;38(3):821-32.

[5] Park YH, Kang H, Woo YC, Park SG, Baek CW, Jung YH, Kim JY, Koo GH, Kim SD, Park JS. The effect of intraperitoneal ropivacaine on pain after laparoscopic colectomy: a prospective randomized controlled trial. *J Surg Res*. 2011; 171(1):94-100.

[6] Di Pace MR, Cimador M, Catalano P, Caruso A, Sergio M, Casuccio A, et al. Efficacy of periportal infiltration and intraperitoneal instillation of ropivacaine after laparoscopic surgery in children. *J Laparoendosc Adv Surg Tech A*. 2009;19(6):821-5.

[7] Makin E, Cross K, Curry J. Regarding: Efficacy of periportal infiltration and intraperitoneal instillation of ropivacaine after laparoscopic surgery in children. *J Laparoendosc Adv Surg Tech A*. 2009; 19(6):845.

[8] Kaufman Y, Hirsch I, Ostrovsky L, Klein O, Shnaider I, Khoury E, et al. Pain relief by continuous intraperitoneal nebulization of ropivacaine during gynecologic laparoscopic surgery--a randomized study and review of the literature. *J Minim Invasive Gynecol.* 2008;15(5):554-8.

[9] Paech MJ, Ilett KF, Hackett LP, Page-Sharp M, Parsons RW. Disposition and clinical outcome after intraperitoneal meperidine and ropivacaine administration during laparoscopic surgery. *Anesth Analg.* 2008; 106(1):278-86.

[10] Ruiz-Tovar J, Gonzalez J, Garcia A, Cruz C, Rivas S, Jimenez M, et al. Intraperitoneal Ropivacaine Irrigation in Patients Undergoing Bariatric Surgery: a Prospective Randomized Clinical Trial. *Obes Surg.* 2016; 26(11):2616-2621.

[11] Tian X, Yang P, Su T, Yu J, Zhao S, Xiang G, et al. Intraperitoneal ropivacaine and early postoperative pain and postsurgical outcomes after laparoscopic herniorrhaphy in toddlers: a randomized clinical trial. *Paediatr Anaesth.* 2016; 26(9):891-8.

[12] Saccardi C, Gizzo S, Vitagliano A, Noventa M, Micaglio M, Parotto M, et al. Peri-incisional and intraperitoneal ropivacaine administration: a new effective tool in pain control after laparoscopic surgery in gynecology: a randomized controlled clinical trial. *Surg Endosc.* 2016; 30(12):5310-5318.

[13] McClure JH. Ropivacaine. *Br J Anaesth.* 1995;76:300–7.

[14] Hansen TG. Ropivacaine: A pharmacological review. *Expert Rev Neurother.* 2004;4:781–91.

[15] Kindler CH, Paul M, Zou H, Liu C, Winegar BD, Gray AT, et al. Amide local anaesthetics potently inhibit the human tandem pore domain background K+ channel TASK-2 (KCNK5) *J Pharmacol Exp Ther.* 2003;306:84–92.

[16] Knudsen K, Beckman Suurküla M, Blomberg S, Sjövall J, Edvardsson N. Central nervous and cardiovascular effects of i.v infusions of ropivacaine, bupivacaine and placebo in volunteers. *Br J Anaesth.* 1997;78:507–14.

[17] Graf BM, Abraham I, Eberbach N, Kunst G, Stowe DF, Martin E. Differences in cardiotoxicity of bupivacaine and ropivacaine are the result of physicochemical and stereoselective properties. *Anesthesiology*. 2002; 96:1427–34.

[18] Graf BM. The cardiotoxicity of local anesthetics: The place of ropivacaine. *Curr Top Med Chem*. 2001; 1:207–14.

[19] Cederholm I, Evers H, Löfström JB. Skin blood flow after intradermal injection of ropivacaine in various concentrations with and without epinephrine evaluated by laser Doppler flowmetry. *Reg Anesth*. 1992; 17:322–8.

[20] Porter J, Crowe B, Cahill M, Shorten G. The effects of ropivacaine hydrochloride on platelet function: An assessment using the platelet function analyser (PFA-100) *Anaesthesia*. 2001; 56:15–8.

[21] Bátai I, Kerényi M, Falvai J, Szabó G. Bacterial growth in ropivacaine hydrochloride. *Anesth Analg*. 2002; 94:729–31.

[22] Kampe S, Poetter C, Buzello S, Wenchel HM, Paul M, Kiencke P, et al. Ropivacaine 0.1% with sufentanil 1 microg/mL inhibits *in vitro*growth of *Pseudomonas aeruginosa* and does not promote multiplication of *Staphylococcus aureus*. *Anesth Analg*. 2003; 97:409–11.

[23] Simpson D, Curran MP, Oldfield V, Keating GM. Ropivacaine: A review of its use in regional anaesthesia and acute pain management. *Drugs*. 2005; 65:2 675–717.

[24] Burm AG, Stienstra R, Brouwer RP, Emanuelsson BM, van Kleef JW. Epidural infusion of ropivacaine for postoperative analgesia after major orthopedic surgery: Pharmacokinetic evaluation. *Anesthesiology*. 2000; 93:395–403.

[25] Ala-Kokko TI, Alahuhta S, Jouppila P, Korpi K, Westerling P, Vähäkangas K. Feto-maternal distribution of ropivacaine and bupivacaine after epidural administration for cesarean section. *Int J Obstet Anesth*. 1997; 6:147–52.

[26] Woolf CJ, Chong MS. Preemptive analgesia – Treating postoperative pain by preventing the establishment of central sensitization. *Anesth Analg* 1993; 77:362-79.

[27] Lee IO, Kim SH, Kong MH, Lee MK, Kim NS, Choi YS, et al. Pain after laparoscopic cholecystectomy: The effect and timing of incisional and intraperitoneal bupivacaine. *Can J Anaesth* 2001; 48:545-50.

[28] Sarac AM, Aktan AO, Baykan N, Yegen C, Yalin R. The effect and timing of local anesthesia in laparoscopic cholecystectomy. *Surg Laparosc Endosc* 1996; 6:362-6.

[29] Barczynski M, Konturek A, Herman RM. Superiority of preemptive analgesia with intraperitoneal instillation of bupivacaine before rather than after the creation of pneumoperitoneum for laparoscopic cholecystectomy: A randomized, double-blind, placebo-controlled study. *Surg Endosc* 2006; 20:1088-93.

[30] Maestroni U, Sortini D, Devito C, Pour Morad Kohan Brunaldi F, Anania G, Pavanelli L, et al. A new method of preemptive analgesia in laparoscopic cholecystectomy. *Surg Endosc* 2002; 16:1336-40.

[31] Bindra TK, Kumar P, Rani P, Kumar A, Bariar H. Preempive analgesia by intraperitoneal instillation of ropivacaine in laparoscopic cholecystectomy. *Anesth Essays Res* 2017; 11:740-4.

[32] Kucuk C, Kadiogullari N, Canoler O, Savli S. A placebo-controlled comparison of bupivacaine and ropivacaine instillation for preventing postoperative pain after laparoscopic cholecystectomy. *Surg Today.* 2007;37(5): 396-400.

[33] Jiménez Fuertes M, Costa Navarro D. Outpatient laparoscopic cholecystectomy and pain control: a series of 100 cases. *Cir Esp.* 2015; 93(3):181-6.

[34] Yong, L, Guang B. Intraperitoneal ropivacaine instillation versus no intraperitoneal ropivacaine instillation for laparoscopic cholecystectomy: A systematic review and meta-analysis. *Int J Surg.* 2017; 44:229-243.

[35] Kahokehr, A, Sammour, T, Soop, M, Hill, AG. Intraperitoneal use of local anesthetic in laparoscopic cholecystectomy: systematic review andmetaanalysis of randomized controlled trials, *J. Hepato-Biliary-Pancreatic Sci.* 17 (5) (2010) 637e656.

[36] Boddy, AP, Mehta, S, Rhodes, M. The effect of intraperitoneal local anesthesia in laparoscopic cholecystectomy: a systematic review and meta-analysis, *Anesth. Analg.* 103 (3) (2006) 682e688.

[37] Choi GJ, Kang H, Baek CW, Jung YH, Kim DR. Effect of intraperitoneal local anesthetic on pain characteristics after laparoscopic cholecystectomy. *World J Gastroenterol.* 2015; 21:13386–13395.

[38] Bucciero M, Ingelmo PM, Fumagalli R, Noll E, Garbagnati A, Somaini M, Joshi GP, Vitale G, Giardini V, Diemunsch P. Intraperitoneal ropivacaine nebulization for pain management after laparoscopic cholecystectomy: a comparison with intraperitoneal instillation. *Anesth Analg.* 2011; 113:1266–1271.

[39] Ahn Y, Woods J, Connor S. *A systematic review of interventions to facilitate ambulatory laparoscopic cholecystectomy.* HPB (Oxford). 2011; 13:677–686.

[40] Kaushal-Deep SM, Anees A, Khan S, Khan MA, Lodhi M. Randomized controlled study of intraincisional infiltration versus intraperitoneal instillation of standardized dose of ropivacaine 0.2% in post-laparoscopic cholecystectomy pain: Do we really need high doses of local anesthetics-time to rethink! *Surg Endosc.* 2018 Jan 16.

[41] Bucciero M, Ingelmo PM, Fumagalli R, et al. Intraperitoneal ropivacaine nebulization for pain management after laparoscopic cholecystectomy: a comparison with intraperitoneal instillation. *Anesth Analg* 2011; 113: 1266–71.

[42] Schlotterbeck H, Schaeffer R, Dow WA, Diemunsch P. Cold nebulization used to prevent heat loss during laparoscopic surgery: an experimental study in pigs. *Surg Endosc* 2008; 22: 2616–20.

[43] Greib N, Schlotterbeck H, Dow WA, Joshi GP, Geny B, Diemunsch PA. An evaluation of gas humidifying devices as a means of intraperitoneal local anesthetic administration for laparoscopic surgery. *Anesth Analg* 2008; 107: 549–51.

[44] Alkhamesi NA, Peck DH, Lomax D, Darzi AW. Intraperitoneal aerosolization of bupivacaine reduces postoperative pain in

laparoscopic surgery: a randomized prospective controlled double-blind clinical trial. *Surg Endosc* 2007; 21: 602–6.

[45] Zimmer PW, McCann MJ, O'Brien MM. Bupivacaine use in the Insuflow device during laparoscopic cholecystectomy: results of a prospective randomized double-blind controlled trial. *Surg Endosc* 2010; 24: 1524–7.

[46] Betton D, Greib N, Schlotterbeck H, Joshi G, Ubeaud-Sequier G, Diemunsch P. The pharmacokinetics of ropivacaine after intra-peritoneal administration: instillation versus nebulization. *Anesth Analg* 2010; 111: 1140–5.

[47] Ingelmo PM, Bucciero M, Somaini M, Sahillioglu E, Garbagnati A, Charton A et al. Intraperitoneal nebulization of ropivacaine for pain control after laparoscopic cholecystectomy: a double-blind, randomized, placebo-controlled trial. *Br J Anaesth*. 2013; 110 (5):800-6.

In: Management of Postoperative Pain ... ISBN: 978-1-53614-284-6
Editor: Jaime Ruiz-Tovar

Chapter 9

PERITONEAL LAVAGE AND LAPAROSCOPIC SLEEVE GASTRECTOMY SURGERY

Lorea Zubiaga*[1,*]*, MD, PhD
and Jaime Ruiz-Tovar*[2]*, MD, PhD
[1]Inserm, Lille 2 University, Lille, France
[2]Surgery Department, Autonoma University, Madrid, Spain

ABSTRACT

To prevent or remove bacterial proliferation after different abdominal surgeries, different solutions for peritoneal lavage have been proposed. This procedure is usually described on laparotomic surgery, but it is not current practice on laparoscopic procedures. Peritoneal lavage may reduce bacterial contamination, but does not completely eliminate them. The addition of antibiotic agents might further reduce the bacterial contamination. Despite surgical-site infection is a relatively rare complication after bariatric surgery, antibiotic lavage does not show its effect on this issue. However, the eventual reduction in the bacterial contamination reduces the inflammatory response and consequently diminishes the postoperative pain.

[*] Corresponding Author Email: loreazubiaga@gmail.com.

Keywords: peritoneal lavage, antibiotic solution, postoperative pain, acute-phase reactants, peritoneal contamination, surgical site infection

INTRODUCTION

Following laparotomy, abdominal surgery develops some degree of peritoneal contamination and surgical site infection (SSI) due to complex processes involving injured tissues and peritoneum. For most patients, peritoneal contamination and SSI have no clinical consequences due to the effectiveness of the patient's own immune response and prophylaxis with intravenous antibiotics, but SSI is associated with increased health care resource utilization and, in some cases, the peritoneal contamination is the prelude to infectious problems that go unnoticed until it is too late. [1] It is assumed that many of these processes of SSI have been significantly reduced by the shift from conventional laparotomy to laparoscopic surgery. [2]

Surgical site infection (SSI) is one of the most common complications of abdominal surgery. It is associated with longer hospital stays, lower quality of life and increased morbidity and mortality and sanitary cost. Centers for disease control (CDC) defines SSI as infection that occurs in or near the surgical incision during the first 30 days, or up to one year, if an implant has been left in place. [3] SSI occurs when the bacterial inoculum exceeds the ability of the immune system to control it. Contamination in abdominal surgery comes from the skin or target organs being treated. The abdominal organs are typically the gastrointestinal tract, a system that coexists with a significant number of microbes that under normal conditions are contained by the immune system, but in cases of surgical aggression can become highly virulent pathogens.

The determinants of infection are the surgeon, the pathogen and the patient. [3, 4] The surgeon is the main modulator of the surgical infection. Their experience and ability can reduce the inoculum to dimensions controllable by the body's defenses. A proper surgical procedure includes careful tissue management, good hemostasis, no unnecessary lengthening of surgical time and minimizing extravasation of gastrointestinal contents. Patients´ dependent factors include comorbidities, obesity, smoking, and old age.

Many surgeons have adopted peritoneal lavage on different abdominal surgeries, mainly by laparotomy and/or peritonitis conditions. [5] This lavage usually consists of peritoneal irrigation with a variable volume of warm 0.9% sodium chloride physiologic solution (Saline Solution –SS-). The main mechanism of action of these lavages is to remove large accumulations of infectious material (feces, pus, necrotic tissue, etc.) and to dilute as much as possible the bacterial charge and other materials, that promote bacterial proliferation (e.g., blood) at the peritoneum. However, the effects of lavage have been widely studied, but with controversial results yet. [5-7] Peritoneal lavage can be altered by three basic variables: volume of irrigation fluid, timing of delivery and/or solution composition. Therefore, flushing the peritoneal cavity may also reduce the bacterial load and possibly minimize the risk of SSI. [8] Obviously, the efficacy of peritoneal irrigations in peritonitis is unclear. Moreover, the prophylactic effect of lavage in elective clean contaminated surgery is even less well understood than in peritonitis, because few relevant studies have been conducted.

Cases of undiagnosed serious abdominal infections are also common in obese patients undergoing bariatric surgery, as in many cases they are patients with a series of comorbidities (such as diabetes and dyslipemia) that aggravate the basal situation. [9] Gastric leak after sleeve gastrectomy is associated with significant and prolonged morbidity, remaining one of the most feared complications. Based on the data from International Sleeve Gastrectomy Expert Panel Consensus Statement 2011, the leak rate was near to 1.06%, but the leak rate can vary between 1% and 3% for primary procedure and more than 10% in revision techniques. [10] A gastric leak can present as peritonitis, abscesses, cutaneous or other fistulas, sepsis, organ failure and even death.

Furthermore performing a lavage with large amounts of SS is not a frequent procedure in laparoscopic bariatric surgery, since achieving the total and correct aspiration of all the infused serum is not easy in obese patients. The obese patients have an important amount of visceral adipose tissue, which makes any maneuver in the abdominal cavity even more difficult. Above all, it is precisely the visceral fat of obese patients that has a high capacity to hide the bacterial niches and reproduce process of infection, which are difficult to diagnose and treat. For this reason, it has been proposed to use antibiotic solutions for the peritoneal lavage.

Peritoneal Lavage with Antibiotic Solutions

Several antibiotics have been used for peritoneal lavage in diverse pathologies. The most widely investigated pathologies, in which antibiotic solutions were used was peritonitis. [8, 11] Up to our knowledge, our group was the first one to investigate the effect of peritoneal lavage with antibiotic solutions in bariatric surgery. We evaluated the effects of peritoneal lavage with physiologic saline solution (SS) or an antibiotic solution (AS) (clindamycin–gentamicin) on post-operative pain, acute-phase reactants and SSI. The microbiologic impact of both irrigations on peritoneal contamination was also determined.

A randomized study was performed with the following inclusion criteria were body mass index (BMI) either >40kg/m2 or >35kg/m2 with co-morbidities associated with obesity and undergoing laparoscopic sleeve gastrectomy (LSG) as a bariatric procedure. Exclusion criteria were documented uncontrolled psychiatric disorders, active infection or malignant disease, gastroesophageal reflux and other concomitant pathologies considered to be a contraindication to perform the LSG. A pre-operative diagnosis of chronic renal failure (because of the risk of nephrotoxicity associated with intraperitoneal gentamicin absorption) was also considered an exclusion criterion.

The surgical technique was performed as usual for LSG: A longitudinal resection from the angle of His to approximately 3 to 4 cm cranially to the pylorus was performed using a 40 French bougie inserted along the lesser curve. A staple line inversion was performed with a continuous over-sewing of polypropylene 3-0 before extracting the bougie.

The remnant stomach was extracted through the 12-mm port site located in the right hypochondrium. The aponeurotic defect of only the 12-mm port site was closed using two simple sutures of poly-dioxanone (size 2) and the skin of all port sites with staples.

The lavage was performed with an irrigation-aspiration device immediately prior to closure of the port sites. In Group 1, irrigation of the entire abdominal cavity was performed with 500 mL of SS. In Group 2, lavage was carried out with the AS, including gentamicin (240 mg) and clindamycin (600mg) dissolved in 500mL of physiologic saline. In both groups, the solution was allowed to stand in the abdominal cavity for 3 min. Pre-operative systemic prophylaxis was performed in all the patients with cefazoline 3g intravenously and another dose of cefazoline.

Prior to any lavage, a microbiologic sample was obtained from the peritoneal surface (parietal and visceral from the gastric tube) with a swab introduced through the 12-mm port site (sample 1). After the assigned lavage and aspiration of the irrigation liquid, a new microbiologic sample was obtained from the peritoneum and the visceral surface of the gastric tube (sample 2). The drainage volume on the second day was collected in a syringe for microbiologic study (sample 3).

Table 1. Baseline features of the patients

	SS	**AS**	**P**
N	40	40	
Mean Age (±SD)	41.6 ±7.1	44.6 ±7.4	0.541
BMI (±SD)	46.9 ±7.5	48.7 ±7.6	0.732
Female/male	30/10	32/8	0.689
Comorbidities (%)			
T2D	8 (20)	9 (22.5)	0.781
Hypertension	10 (25)	10 (25)	1
Dyslipidemia	7 (17.5)	8 (20)	0.772
SAHS	6(15)	5 (12.5)	0.745

(SS: Saline Solution; AS: Antibiotic Solution; SD: Standard Deviation; BMI: Body Mass Index; T2D: Type 2 Diabetes; SAHS: sleep apnea/hypopnea syndrome).

The clinical variables investigated were age, gender, co-morbidities, complications (gastric leak, incisional SSI, and organ-space SSI), post-operative pain assessed 24 hours after surgery by the Visual Analog Scale for Pain (VAS) and morphine needs, occurrence of post- operative nausea or vomiting, analytical variables determined 24 hours after surgery (C-reactive protein [CRP]; white blood cell [WBC] count and lactic acid) compared to hospital stay. Microbiologic variables consisted of cultures of the three extracted samples.

Incisional SSI was defined as the presence of a purulent discharge from any of the surgical sites confirmed with culture. An epidemiology nurse blinded to the treatment groups determined incisional SSI. Infection surveillance was extended for 30 days after discharge. Organ-space SSI was defined as a fluid collection on a contrast-enhanced computed tomography (CT) scan in a patient presenting with fever, tachycardia, abdominal pain, or septic status. The evidence of oral contrast extravasation on a CT scan was considered a leak rather than an organ-space SSI. A radiologist blinded to the treatment group determined the diagnosis of organ-space SSI and leak in case there was one.

A total of 80 patients were included in the study, 40 in each group. The sample consisted of 62 females and 18 males with a mean age of 43 ± 7.2 years. Pre-operative BMI of 47.8 Kg/m^2 ± 7.7 Kg/m^2. The distribution of age, gender, BMI, and co-morbidities was similar in both groups (Table 1).

The post-operative complication rate was 3.7%, consisting of two leaks at the Hiss angle junction (one in each group), satisfactorily resolved with conservative treatment. In SS group one deceased occurred due to pulmonary embolism despite correct thromboembolic prophylaxis. There were no significant differences in the morbidity or mortality rates in the two groups. Given that the hospital stay, pain perception, and laboratory values of the three patients presenting with complications might be altered, as intra-abdominal infection can lead to elevation of all of them, these patients were excluded from the analysis of post- operative pain, laboratory values of acute-phase reactants, and microbiologic study.

The median post-operative pain score 24 hours after surgery was 3.5 (range 2–7) in Group SS and 1.5 (range 0–4) in Group AS ($p = 0.021$).

Morphine administration was required in two patients in Group SS and 0 in Group AS (p = 0.15). Post-operative nausea or vomiting appeared in five patients (13%) in Group AS and 4 (10%) in Group SS (p = 0.72).

The laboratory data 24 hours after surgery are shown in the graphic below (Figure 1). The WBC count also was significantly higher in Group SS (mean difference 1,930/mm3; 95% CI 145–66,839; p = 0.029). The mean CRP concentration also was higher in Group SS (mean difference 27.3 mg/L; 95% CI 16.4–71.2; p = 0.036). Finally, the mean lactic acid concentration also was higher in Group SS (mean difference 0.34 mg/L; 95% CI 0.1–0.7; p = 0.049). The median hospital stay was 3.5 days (range 3–5 days) in Group SS and 2.5 days (range 2–4 days) in Group AS (p = 0.05).

The culture of sample 1 (before any lavage) was positive in seven cases (18.4%) in Group SS and eight cases (20.5%) in Group AS (p = 0.77). The culture of sample 2 (after lavage) was positive in 18.4% of the patients in Group SS and 0 in Group AS (p = 0.006). The culture of sample 3 (drainage discharge) was positive in three patients (7.9%) in Group SS and 0 in Group AS (p = 0.08). The microorganism detected was *Escherichia coli* in all cases. No significant association between microbiologic contamination and clinical or analytical variables could be demonstrated.

In case of peritonitis a peritoneal lavage is mandatory to obtain prompt and fast resolution of the severe infection. [6] In fact, the ideal peritoneal lavage solution should be effective, easy to apply and with low posterior complications or adhesions formation. Several studies tried to establish effective protocols of peritoneal lavage; some authors focused on the effect of temperature, the volume of solution or different methods, such as cyclic intraperitoneal lavage by bi-luminal drainages. Meanwhile, no method has been universally accepted yet. [12] Some authors showed that peritoneal lavage with saline, antibiotics, or antiseptics solution does not influence the outcome following laparotomies for peritonitis. Having so few conclusions in laparotomic surgery, it is evident that much less evidence exists in laparoscopic one. [1]

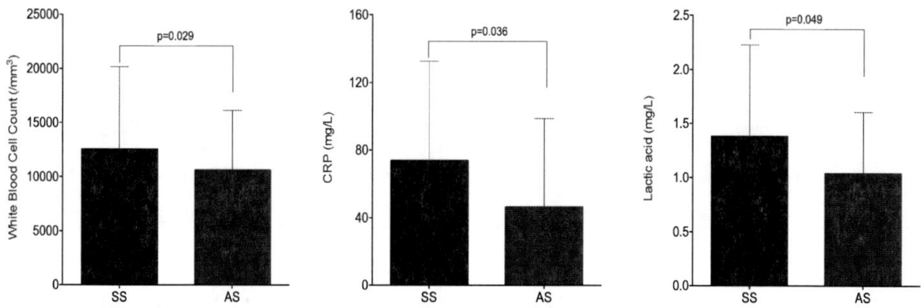

Figure 1. Laboratory data 24 hours after surgery

The LSG is considered a clean-contaminated procedure, because the stomach is divided during this procedure. Thus, peri-operative systemic antibiotic prophylaxis is usually administered. In this sense, the SSI rate after laparoscopic surgery is significantly lower than that after conventional surgery, and this is especially relevant in morbidly obese subjects, as this condition itself is a risk factor for post-operative SSI. In this study, the highest contamination rate was 20% in both groups and the only micro-organism that grew in the cultures was *E. coli*. Thus, the peritoneal contamination in laparoscopically performed operations is much lower than conventional open surgeries and not only reduces the incisional SSI. [9] The abdominal wound is an important problem in obese patients, not only by the size of the skin-peritoneum damage, but also as the subcutaneous fatty tissue is easily colonized by skin flora. It is evident that laparoscopy must be the elective approach for obese patients. In this way, the contamination of SSI is reduced to the intestinal saprophytic flora in the peritoneum and contamination of the subcutaneous tissue is avoided.

The concept of antibiotic irrigation is focused on reduction of SSI on wound. It seems to make no sense when performed in patients undergoing laparoscopic bariatric surgery with such a low contamination rate compared with colorectal surgery. [11] The fact that, SSI rates are not as high as in contaminated procedures reveals that host immunity can control contamination in most cases. The host as an aggression identifies the microorganism contamination, and it produces an inflammatory response. Surgical dissection indeed is an aggression sufficient to start an inflammatory response, but bacterial contamination might contribute to the increase and prolong it. [5]

Among several markers of inflammation, CRP has been studied widely to investigate its accuracy for the diagnosis of bacterial infection and the associated inflammatory response. [14, 15] The protein is an acute-phase reactant, synthesized by the liver, mainly in response to interleukin-6, which is produced not only during infection, but also in many types of inflammation, including the normal course after open or laparoscopic abdominal surgery. This fact justifies the higher concentrations of CRP observed in the post-operative course of most patients, even those having uncomplicated surgery. [14] Furthermore, CRP elevation is predictive of infective post-operative complications. In our series, the elevated CRP concentrations were markers of greater contamination. [16]

For fibrinogen, we could not find an effect like that reported for other acute-phase reactants. However, the accuracy of fibrinogen measurement for the diagnosis of inflammatory response secondary to bacterial infection or contamination seems to be lower, as reported by other authors. [17, 18]

Post-operative pain is a clinical reflection of tissue damage and the consequent inflammatory response. Local release of cytokines by the inflammatory cells stimulates nociceptive nervous receptors, and these trigger pain perception. Thus, a greater inflammatory response increases pain. After surgery the pain perception evaluated by VAS correlates directly with inflammatory cytokines concentrations. [19] In the present study, we could not demonstrate any association between pain, analytical values, and contamination. However, the reduction of all these parameters in the group of patients, who underwent antibiotic irrigation, indicates that the clinical relevance of these procedures beyond the improvement of acute-phase reactants is the reduction of post-operative pain. [20]

According to the results obtained, we believe that peritoneal lavage with antibiotic solution can be recommended in patients undergoing laparoscopic sleeve gastrectomy, and probably other bariatric procedures, but the latter hypothesis must be confirmed in similar studies conducted in other bariatric operations. Another limitation of this study is the small sample, which we used in order to obtain significant results on SSI reduction, one of the principal objectives of the study. More studies must be conducted with larger samples to confirm these hypotheses.

CONCLUSION

Intraperitoneal irrigation with a gentamicin and clindamycin solution in patients undergoing LSG leads to less alteration of acute-phase reactants, decrease postoperative pain and shorter hospital stay. Peritoneal lavage with antibiotic solutions can be considered an effective tool in the multimodal analgesia for bariatric surgery.

REFERENCES

[1] Chopra T. Epidemiology and outcomes associated with surgical site infection following bariatric surgery. *Am J Infect Control* 2012;40(9)(2012):815-9.

[2] Markides G. Laparoscopic versus open appendectomy in adults with complicated appendicitis: systematic review and meta-analysis." *World J Surg* 2010;34(9):2026-40.

[3] Henriksen NA. Clinical relevance of surgical site infection as defined by the criteria of the Centers for Disease Control and Prevention. *J Hosp Infect* 2010;75(3):173-7.

[4] Norman G. Intracavity lavage and wound irrigation for prevention of surgical site infection. *Cochrane Database Syst Rev.* 2017: CD012234.

[5] Qadan M. Meta-analysis of the effect of peritoneal lavage on survival in experimental peritonitis. *Br J Surg* 2010; 97(2):151-9.

[6] Platell C. The influence of lavage on peritonitis. *J Am Coll Surg* 2010;191:672–80.

[7] Adam U. Programmed lavage as a basic principle in therapy of diffuse peritonitis. *Langenbecks Arch Surg* 1997; 382:S18-21.

[8] Edmiston CE. Intra-Operative Surgical Irrigation of the Surgical Incision: What Does the Future Hold-Saline, Antibiotic Agents, or Antiseptic Agents? *Surg Infect (Larchmt)* 2016; 17(6):656-664.

[9] Doyle SL. Obesity and post-operative complications in patients undergoing non-bariatric surgery. *Obes Rev* 2010;11(12):875-86.

[10] Rosenthal RJ. Sleeve Gastrectomy Expert Panel. International Sleeve Gastrectomy Expert Panel Consensus Statement: best practice guidelines based on experience of >12,000 cases. *Surg Obes Relat Dis* 2012;8(1):8-19.

[11] Ruiz-Tovar J. Effect of peritoneal lavage with clindamycin-gentamicin solution on infections after elective colorectal cancer surgery. *J Am Coll Surg* 2012; 214(2):202-7.

[12] Sortini D. Role of peritoneal lavage in adhesion formation and survival rate in rats: an experimental study. *J Invest Surg* 2006; 19(5):291-7.

[13] Ruiz-Tovar, J. Prevention of surgical site infection in abdominal surgery. A critical review of the evidence. *Cir Esp* 2014; 92(4):223 31.

[14] Muñoz JL. C-Reactive Protein and Procalcitonin as Early Markers of Septic Complications after Laparoscopic Sleeve Gastrectomy in Morbidly Obese Patients Within an Enhanced Recovery After Surgery Program. *J Am Coll Surg* 2016; 222(5):831-7.

[15] Woeste G. Increased serum levels of C-reactive protein precede anastomotic leakage in colorectal surgery. *World J Surg* 2010; 34:140-6.

[16] Welsch T. C-reactive protein as early predictor for infectious postoperative complications in rectal surgery. *Int J Colorectal Dis* 2007; 22:1499–507.

[17] Feng S. Hyperfibrinogenemia in appendicitis: a new predictor of perforation in children. *Pediatr Surg Int* 2014; 30(11):1143-7.

[18] Glantzounis GK. Laparoscopic surgery-induced changes in oxidative stress markers in human plasma. *Surg Endosc* 2001; 15:1315–9.

[19] Ruiz-Tovar J. Evaluation of postoperative pain after laparoscopic cholecystectomy: Correlation between visual analogic scale (VAS)

and systemic stress markers determined in a routine blood analysis. *Surg Chron* 2013;18:209–12.

[20] Ruiz-Tovar J. Effect of Peritoneal Lavage with Clindamycin-Gentamicin Solution on Post-Operative Pain and Analytic Acute-Phase Reactants after Laparoscopic Sleeve Gastrectomy. *Surg Infect (Larchmt)* 2016; 17(3):357-62.

In: Management of Postoperative Pain … ISBN: 978-1-53614-284-6
Editor: Jaime Ruiz-Tovar

Chapter 10

IMMUNOMODULATORS AND POSTOPERATIVE PAIN: IMMUNONUTRITION AND TOPICAL VITAMIN E

Jaime Ruiz-Tovar*[1,*]*, MD, PhD
and Carolina Llavero*[2]*,
[1]Department of Surgery,
Universidad Autonoma de Madrid, Spain
[2]Department of Surgical Nursery,
Garcilaso Clinic, Madrid, Spain

ABSTRACT

Immunomodulating agents are involved in regulating the inflammatory response against a surgical damage. The release of proinflammatory agents leads to an increase postoperative pain. Thus, the use of immunomodulating agents, avoiding an excessive production of proinflammatory cytokines, can help to achieve a better control of postoperative pain.

---

* Corresponding Author Email: jruiztovar@gmail.com.

Among the immunomodulating agents, vitamin E and the components of immunonutrition (Omega-3 fatty acids, glutamin, arginin, nucleic acids and antioxidant agents) have been the most widely investigated. The actual evidence of their use in bariatric surgery for postoperative pain control will be discussed in this chapter.

Keywords: pain, bariatric surgery, immunonutrition, vitamin E

IMMUNONUTRITION

Classically, nutritional supplements were focused on reversing the deficiencies in order to achieve sufficient substrate to start the immune machinery. However, research into specific nutritional components that may favorably affect immune function has stimulated the development of enteral products designed to improve the outcomes of hospitalized patients by reducing infections or modulating the inflammatory response to a damage. This way developed the concept of "Immunonutrition." The term "Immunonutrition" (IMN) describes the enteral administration of certain substrates (arginine, omega-3 fatty acids, nucleotides, glutamine and antioxidants) with a putative immunomodulating function. Animal models and human studies have suggested that the individual components have beneficial (or potentially beneficial) effects on immune function.

Components of Immunonutrition

Arginine

Arginine is an essential amino acid because endogenous production may be inadequate during periods of illness or injury. Supplemental arginine seems to improve nitrogen balance, increases T-cell function and stimulates wound healing by favoring collagen deposits.

Oncologic patients who received supplemental arginine showed significant improvement in T-lymphocyte response and increase of CD4-T-cells population.

Arginine is a substrate for production of nitric oxide. Arginase and nitric oxide synthase compete for arginine as a substrate, and the metabolic products of these enzymes are important modulators of T-cell function.

Glutamine

Glutamine is an amino acid with important oxidative function in the cell division, including enterocytes and colonocytes. Glutamine also serves as a nitrogen shuttle and gluconeogenic precursor in the Cori cycle, and as a primary component of the antioxidant glutathione.

Several studies have shown that those patients who received parenteral nutrition supplemented with glutamine, presented lower infection rates.

Omega-3 Fatty Acids

Fish oils are rich in the omega-3 fatty acids eicosapentanoic acid (EPA) and docosahexaenoic acid (DHA). These fatty acids compete with arachadonic acid (omega-6) and participate in the synthesis of prostaglandins, leukotrienes, thromboxanes and prostacyclins. The addition of EPA and DHA to enteral nutrition products results in a reduction of proinflammatory mediators. The addition of omega-3 fatty acids to nutritional supplements have been associated with reduced infectious complications.

Marine sources of omega-3 fats can increase the generation of free radicals and increase apparent antioxidant requirements.

Nucleotides

The normal diet provides 1–2 grams of nucleotides per day from animal proteins, peas, beans, and milk. However, most enteral supplements lack of preformed nucleotides. Animal models fed with a nucleotide-free diet demonstrate an impaired immune response and decreased survival in response to infection.

Antioxidants

One component of IMN formulas that should not be overlooked is the increased amounts of vitamin E, vitamin C, selenium and zinc. There are increasing data that antioxidant vitamins and minerals may positively influence outcome in critically ill patients. A recent study in critically ill surgical patients reported that patients who received vitamin C and E supplements had reduced pulmonary morbidity and the incidence of multi-organ failure. The isolated effect of Vitamin E will be discussed elsewhere.

Only one meta-analysis addressed the clinical importance of a selective antioxidant therapy. It was concluded that such a therapy lowered mortality rates by about one third. However, this effect was unrelated to an improvement of infectious morbidity. Still, parenteral antioxidant supplementation (especially of selenium) is currently considered beneficial in critically ill patients.

Effects of Inmmunonutrition on Postoperative Pain After Bariatric Surgery

Most of the reported evidence of IMN in surgical patients has been focused on malignant pathologies, reporting decreases in postoperative complications and mainly in surgical site infections. Little has been published about the effect of IMN on morbidly obese patients undergoing bariatric surgery. Our group developed a study investigating the effect of IMN on patients undergoing laparoscopic sleeve gastrectomy. Given that in bariatric surgery the incidence of complications is relative small, especially infectious complications, we analyzed postoperative pain and analytic acute-phase reactants as markers of the surgical aggression, trying to elucidate if the immunomodulating effect of IMN would have some effect on these parameters. As expected, the patients receiving IMN two weeks before surgery presented lower postoperative pain and lower values of C reactive protein. Clinically, the anti-inflammatory effect can be represented as a reduction in the postoperative. Though CRP is a relatively weak inflammatory indicator, it is easy to evaluate clinically, as it is an available parameter in a routine blood analysis. Surgery stimulates a series of hormonal and metabolic changes that constitute the stress response. It has been demonstrated that stress response is associated with the postoperative pain feeling. Proinflammatory parameters, such as

Interleukin-6 (IL-6) and TNF-α, have been involved in the response to the surgical aggression.

Surprisingly, a reduction in liver enzymes was also observed in our study. Another publication of our group revealed that postoperative pain shows a significant correlation with transaminase levels (AST and ALT) in plasma after laparoscopic cholecystectomy. Previous studies have shown that laparoscopic surgery causes transient hepatic hypoperfusion secondary to a blood flow reduction, damaging the hepatocelular integrity and causing an increase of plasma levels of liver enzymes. This finding was attributed to the combined effects of elevated intra-abdominal pressure, hypercapnia and the position of the patient. Humoral factors, such as vasopressin released from the pituitary during the surgical act, may also be involved in hepatic blood flow during laparoscopic surgery. Other possible hypothesis to justify the significantly lower levels of postoperative transaminases might be a reduction in the Non-Alcoholic Fatty Liver Disease (NAFLD). NAFLD includes a spectrum of disorders ranging from simple steatosis, a relatively benign condition, to nonalcoholic steato-hepatitis (NASH) and pericellular or perisinusoidal fibrosis. The prevalence of NAFLD in any degree, is estimated in up to 95% in morbidly obese patients. Among patients undergoing bariatric surgery, liver steatosis is the most common degree of the disease, but Non-Alcoholic Steatohepatitis (NASH) appears in about 25% of the cases. IMN and its immunomodulating effect might probably reduce the inflammatory response to the lipid deposit in the hepatocytes of the liver parenchyma and thereby the associated hepatitis and hepatolysis.

From all the elements conforming these IMN formulas, Omega-3 Fatty Acids (O3FA) are hypothesized to be the most important component for immunomodulation, with increased antioxidant effect. Thus, we recently conducted a randomized clinical trial, evaluating the effect of isolated O3FA on postoperative pain and analytical acute phase reactants in morbidly obese patients undergoing Roux-en-Y gastric bypass. The results we obtained also demonstrated a reduction in postoperative weight loss and C-reactive protein, similarly to that observed in the previous study with all the components of IMN.

Itariu et al. published in 2012 a study, analyzing the effect of the administration of long-chain n3- polyunsaturated fatty acids (EPA and DHA) for 8 weeks in morbidly obese patients before undergoing bariatric surgery on inflammatory gene expressions in visceral and subcutaneous fat. They observed that, in patients receiving EPA and DHA, the inflammatory genes expression and the circulating levels of IL-6 were decreased. Ianelly et al. evaluated the effect of a preoperative 4-week supplementation with omega-3 polyunsaturated fatty acids on the liver volume, determining a 20% reduction of the volume of the left hepatic lobe. These authors did not attribute the decrease of the liver volume to weight loss, as they did not establish any preoperative dietary restriction for these patients. Abidin et al. examined liver volume by MRI and body weight of bariatric candidates after 4 weeks of preoperative treatment with a very low calorie diet (VLCD) or with 2000 mg/day omega 3, without dietary restriction and they found that omega 3 supplementation (without dietary restriction) had the same effect in reducing liver volume and body weight as did the VLCD.

Both of our studies are not comparable, because the surgical techniques were different, so that we cannot conclude that the same benefit is obtained with only O3FA, when compared with the addition of arginine, glutamine and nucleic acids. As previously mentioned, all the components of IMN have a certain inmmunomodulating function, but in our opinion the addition of all has probably a synergistic effect.

TOPICAL VITAMIN E

Topical application of vitamin E ointment has demonstrated a certain anti-inflammatory effect in dermatologic diseases. Vitamin E achieves a reduction of edema and moderates the increase of cyclooxigenase-2 (COX-2), an enzyme that catalyzes the synthesis of prostaglandin E2, involved in the local inflammatory response against aggression. Vitamin E has been also widely used in gynaecological disorders, mainly affecting the vulvar skin and vaginal mucosae. Postoperatively, vitamin is used with cosmetic effect, as the reduction of the local inflammatory response is associated with an enlarged scar. Moreover, it has been demonstrated that vitamin E is also associated with a reduction in postoperative pain of skin wounds. Immunomodulation effect of vitamin E affects humoral and cell-mediated immune responses. Vitamin E has demonstrated to modulate the neutrophils recruitment to the damaged tissue.

Postoperative pain is a multifactorial complication, depending on the individual tolerance, mode of anesthesia, postoperative analgesics and aggressiveness of the surgical act. Alleviation of pain should be achieved by minimizing tissue dissection and using carefully the electrosurgical devices to diminish thermal injury to the subjacent tissues. However, the application of local substances can be helpful to reduce the pain sensation. Topical drugs employed can be local anesthetics, but it has been widely demonstrated that their effect is transitory and the pain peak often appears after the first 24 hours postoperatively, just coinciding with the highest point of inflammatory response of the organism. Thus, actually several immunomodulating agents are investigated with the aim of reducing the postoperative response against the surgical damage.

In this line, vitamin E is natural active principle, without associating adverse effects. Our group has used topical vitamin E acetate in the surgical bed of hemorrhoidectomy and has obtained extraordinary results, probably based on a reduction in the local inflammatory response against surgical aggression due to its anti-inflammatory effect. The clinical reflection of this mechanism of action is a significant reduction of postoperative pain, an improvement in quality of life and an earlier reincorporation to normal activities.

Furthermore, a recent study of our group, analyzing the effect of subcutaneous application of sterile vitamin E acetate after laparoscopic colorectal surgery, has shown a reduction in the postoperative surgical site infection (SSI), postoperative pain and analytical acute phase reactants. Local drugs delivery for prevention of incisional SSI was based on application of antibiotics or antiseptics, based on the hypothesis that these agents might reduce the bacterial contamination and consequently reduce the infection rate. However, it is widely known that the three factors participating in the surgical infection are bacterial contamination, surgical team and host. Thus, a different inflammatory response to the local aggression might contribute to the development of SSI, acting the immunomodulating effect of vitamin E as a protective factor against it. Moreover, independently of this immunomodulation, the acetate radical of vitamin E acetate applied in this study might also have bactericidal effect. Acetate radicals have shown to be highly effective against gram-negative microbacteria. The association of Vitamin E ointment with lower acute phase reactants levels reflects that apart from a protective effect against incisional SSI, the immunomodulation induced by Vitamin E reduces the surgical aggression just caused by the surgery, independently of the development of SSI. The clinical translation of this lower inflammatory response induced by vitamin E is the lower pain perception, as measured by VAS 24 hours after laparoscopic colorectal surgery.

Given the excellent results of topical vitamin E on postoperative pain after hemorrhoidectomy and colorectal surgery, we develop a research protocol, to apply topical vitamin E ointment on the staple line and anastomoses of Roux-en-Y gastric bypass. Postoperative pain and acute phase reactants were investigated. As expected, the patients presented a reduction of postoperative pain, as measured by Visual Analogic Scale 24 hours after surgery, and morphine needs during the hospital stay. Laboratory data revealed a reduction in C reactive protein levels and White Blood Cells count. Secondary to the decrease of pain and lowered requirement of opioids, the patients were able to achieve early ambulation and oral intake, finally leading to an early hospital discharge and a lower impact of the surgery on the quality of life.

CONCLUSION

Immunomodulating agents, such as IMN or vitamin E, among others, can be useful weapons for the treatment of postoperative pain after bariatric surgery. They can reduce postoperative discomfort and improve the surgical impact and quality of life in the immediate postoperative course. These measures are used by the surgeon, independently of the analgesic regimen prescribed by the anesthesiologist. Therefore, they can be considered as useful tools in the multimodal approach of postoperative pain, within an Enhanced Recovery After Surgery (ERAS) program.

REFERENCES

Abidin ZAZ, Kosai NR, Taher MM, et al. A randomized controlled trial comparing the use of omega-3 polyinsaturated fatty acidsupplements versus very low calorie dietary restriction in obese Malaysian patients awaiting bariatric surgery. *Ann Laparosc Endosc Surg* 2017;2:112-117.

Alexander JW, Saito H, Trocki O, et al. The importance of lipid type in the diet after burn injury. *Ann Surg* 1986;204:1-8.

Alias D, Ruiz-Tovar J, Moreno A, Manso B, Diaz G, Durán M, García-Olmo D. Effect of subcutaneous sterile vitamin E ointment on incisional surgical site infection after elective laparoscopiccolorectal cancer surgery. *Surg Infect* 2017;18:287-92.

Alves de Carvalho MS, Coelho Cabral P, Kruze Grande de Arruda I, et al. Risk factors associated with hepatic steatosis; a study in patients in the Northeast Brazil. *Nutr Hosp* 2012;27:1344-1350.

Barbul A. Arginine and immune function. *Nutrition*, 1990;6: 53-58.

Bistrian BR, Blackburn GL, Scrimshaw NS, et al. Cellular immunity in semistarved states in hospitalized adults. *Am J Clin Nutr* 1975; 28:1148-1155.

Bistrian BR, Blackburn GL, Vitale J, et al. Prevalence of malnutrition in general medical patients. *JAMA* 1976;235:1567- 1570.

Bou Ghanem EN, Clark S, Du X, et al. The α-tocopherol form of vitamin E reverses age-associated susceptibility to streptococcus pneumoniae lung infection by modulating pulmonary neutrophil recruitment. *J Immunol* 2015; 194:1090-1099.

Bravo-Cuellar A, Romero-Ramos JE, Hernandez-Flores G, et al. Comparación de dos tipos de anestesia en los nive-les plasmáticos de marcadores inflamatorios. *Cir Cir* 2007; 75:99-100. [Comparison of two types of anesthesia in the plasma levels of inflammatory markers.]

Cerantola Y, Hubner M, Grass F, et al. Immunonutrition in gastrointestinal surgery. *Br J Surg* 2011;98:37-48.

Clark JM, Alkhuraishi AR, Solga SF, et al. Roux-en-Y gastric bypass improves liver histology in patients with non-alcoholic fatty liver disease. *Obes Res* 2005;13:1180-1186.

Conforti S, Di Serio C, Cartoccio P, et al. Our experience in the treatment of vulvar sclerous lichen. *Clin Exp Obstet Gynecol* 1988;15:178-180.

Crimi E, Liguori A, Condorelli M, et al. The beneficial effects of antioxidant supplementation in enteral feeding in critically ill patients: a prospective, randomized, double blind, placebo-controlled trial. *Anesth Analg* 2004;99:857-863.

Crimi E, Liguori A, Condorelli M, et al. The beneficial effects of antioxidant supplementation in enteral feeding in critically ill patients: a prospective, randomized, double blind, placebo-controlled trial. *Anesth Analg* 2004;99:857-863.

Daly JM, Reynolds J, Thom A, et al. Immune and metabolic effects of arginine in the surgical patient. *Ann Surg* 1988; 208:512-523.

Freeman LJ, Rahmani EY, Al-Haddad M, et al. Comparison of pain and postoperative stress in dogs undergoing natural orifice transluminal endoscopic surgery, laparoscopic and open oophorectomy. *Gastrointest Endosc* 2010; 72:373-380.

Gach JE, Humphreys F, Berth-Jones J. Randomized, doublé-blind, placebo-controlled pilot study to assess the value of free radical scavengersin reducing inflammation induced by cryotherapy. *Clin Exp Dermatol* 2005; 30: 14-16.

Galban C, Montejo JC, Mesejo A, et al. An immune-enhancing enteral diet reduces mortality rate and episodes of bacteremia in septic intensive care unit patients. *Crit Care Med* 2000; 28:643-648.

Iannelli A, Martini F, Schneck AS, et al. Preoperative 4-week supplementation with omega-3 polyunsaturated fatty acids reduces liver volume and facilitates bariatric surgery in morbidly obese patients. *Obes Surg* 2013; 23:1761-1765.

Itariu BK, Zeyda M, Hochbrugger EE, et al. Long-chain n-3 PUFAs reduce adipose tissue and systemic inflammation in severely obese nondiabetic patients: a randomized controlled trial. *Am J Clin Nutr* 2012;96:1137-1149.

Kelley DS. Modulation of human immune and inflammatory responses by dietary fatty acids. *Nutrition* 2001;17:669- 673.

Kotake Y, Takeda J, Matsumoto M, et al. Subclinical hepatic dysfunction in laparoscopic cholecystectomy and laparoscopic colectomy. *Br J Anaesthesia* 2001; 87:774-777.

Kulkarni AD, Fanslow WC, Drath DB, et al. Influence of dietary nucleotide restriction on bacterial sepsis and phagocytic cell function in mice. *Arch Surg* 1986;121;169-172.

Law DK, Dudrick SJ, Abdou NI. The effects of protein calorie malnutrition on immune competence of the surgical patient. *Surg Gynecol Obstet* 1974;139:257-266.

Nathens AB, Neff MJ, Jurkovich GJ, et al. Randomized, Prospective Trial of Antioxidant Supplementation in Critically Ill Surgical Patients. *Ann Surg* 2002;236:814-822.

Peck MD. Omega-3 polyunsaturated fatty acids: benefit or harm during sepsis? *New Horizons* 1994;2:230-236.

Ruiz-Tovar J, Duran M, Alias D, et al. Reduction of postoperative pain and improvement of patients' comfort after Milligan-Morgan hemorrhoidectomy using topical application of vitamin E ointment. *Int J Colorectal Dis* 2016; 31:1371-1372.

Ruiz-Tovar J, Ortega I, Santos J, et al. Evaluation of postoperative pain after laparoscopic cholecystectomy: correlation between visual analogic scale (VAS) and systemic stress markers determined in a routinary blood analysis. *Surg Chron* 2013; 18: 209-212.

Ruiz-Tovar J, Zubiaga L, Diez M, Murcia A, Boix E, Muñoz JL, Llavero C, OBELCHE. Preoperative regular diet of 900 Kcal/day vs Balanced-Energy high protein formula vs Immunonutrition formula: Effect on preoperative weight loss and postoperative pain, complications and analytical acute phase reactants after laparoscopic sleeve gastrectomy. *Obes Surg* 2016; 26:1221-7.

Souba WW, Smith RJ, Wilmore DW. Glutamine metabolism by the intestinal tract. *JPEN*, 1985; 9:608-617.

Van Buren CT, Kulkarni Ad, Fanslow WC, et al. Dietary nucleotides: a requirement for helper/inducer T-lymphocytes. *Transplantation* 1985;40:694-697.

Viera MH, Amini Sm Konda S, et al. Do postsurgical interventions optimize ultimate scar cosmesis? *G Ital Dermatol Venerol* 2009; 144:243-257.

Wilkins T, Tadkod A, Hepburn I, et al. Nonalcoholic fatty liver disease: diagnosis and management. *Am Fam Physician* 2013;88:35-42.

Yoshida E, WatanabeT, Takata J, et al. Topical application of a novel, hydrophylic gamma-tocopherol derivative reduces photo-inflammation in mice skin. *J Invest Dermatol* 2006;126:1633-1640.

Zhang Y, Gu Y, Guo T, et al. Perioperative immunonutrition for gastrointestinal cancer: a systematic review of randomized controlled trials. *Surg Oncol* 2012; 21:e87-e95.

Ziegler TR, Young LS, Benfell K, et al. Clinical and metabolic efficacy of glutamine-supplemented parenteral nutrition after bone marrow transplantation. A randomized, double-blind, controlled study. *Ann Intern Med,* 1992;116(10):821-828.

In: Management of Postoperative Pain … ISBN: 978-1-53614-284-6
Editor: Jaime Ruiz-Tovar

Chapter 11

INFLUENCE OF ERAS PROTOCOLS ON POSTOPERATIVE PAIN

Pablo Royo Dachary, MD, PhD
and Helen Almeida Ponce, MD
Department of Surgery, University of Zaragoza, Zaragoza, Spain

ABSTRACT

Overcoming surgical pain has always been a milestone for the development of new techniques and it has widened the reach for more complex procedures; in fact, it wasn't until general anesthesia was discovered that surgery could finally start reaching its true potential.

By definition, ERAS protocols assure patients the best evidence based care measures. In this chapter, we analyze the influence of ERAS protocols in postoperative pain, and how this influence helps in reducing postoperative stay, postoperative complications and improving patients' experience of the surgical process.

Keywords: postoperative pain, ERAS protocols

INTRODUCTION

> "The escape from pain in surgical operations is a chimera that we cannot afford to achieve at present. 'Knife' and 'pain' in surgery are words which are always inseparable in the minds of patients, and it´s necessary for surgeons to accept this association"
>
> (Alfred-Armand-Louis-Marie Velpeau, 1839)

Overcoming surgical pain has always been a milestone for the development of new techniques and it has widened the reach for more complex procedures. In fact, it wasn't until general anesthesia was discovered that surgery could finally start reaching its true potential.

How was surgery before effective anesthesia? Nowadays, it's impossible to imagine English hospitals used to place the operating rooms on the last floor of the buildings. A glass roof could provide a good illumination for the surgical field, but it also was useful to isolate the rest of the hospital, from the heartrending screams of the patients who were operated on. Surgeons had to be quick and skillful.

Surgery suffered a great revolution with the discovery of surgical anesthesia. The analgesic effects of opium or poppy were known by ancient civilizations centuries ago, but surgical interventions were still a very traumatic procedure that the patient had to deal with consciously. The discovery of anesthetic gases changed the way surgery was known. The nitrous oxide was discovered by the British chemical Joseph Priestley in 1772, and in 1818 an anonymous note was published pointing that ether inhalation had the same effects than nitrous oxide. The dentist Horace Wells (1815-1848) was the first to use it for therapeutic purposes in 1844, but it was Green Morton (1819-1868), a dentist who attended to *Massachusetts Medical College*, who administered the first anesthesia to a patient in the *Massachusetts General Hospital* in 1846. The patient was operated on to treat a neck vascular tumour by John Collis Warren (1778-1856), chief of Surgery Department. The intervention took place in absolute silence, something never seen before in an operating theater.

The American neurologist James Leonard Corning (1855-1923) was the first to perform a neuraxial block in 1885, when he injected 111mg of cocaine into the epidural space. In 1912, the Spanish military surgeon Fidel Pagés (1886-1923) developed the single injection epidural lumbar anesthesia technique. Although epidural anesthesia is commonly related to labor, nowadays multiple surgical interventions can be performed under its effects, and its use has been spread to the perioperative pain control.

During the XX century, the first anesthesic-based Pain Services, were born. The book *Management of* pain published by John Joseph Bonica (1917-2004) in 1953, stablished the base of modern algesiology. The foundation of this Pain Services was the first recognition of an important problem. Lots of patients suffering from pain, were treated in an incorrect way, and the lack of communication suffered by some specialities, prevented the use of available resources. These Services highlighted the importance of multidisciplinarity for the use of the best medical practice.

Regardless of the historical evolution of the concept and the meaning of the word "pain," there are differences in their consideration according to ethnic groups, cultures and religions. Even the pain itself has a strong psychologic component. Henry Knowles Beecher (1904-1976) was an anesthesist in the *Massachusetts General Hospital*, who realized that soldiers seriously injured in the combat front, reported less pain than patients operated on scheduled interventions in the Hospital. The reason found was that soldiers founded in that pain a way to escape from the front, while hospital patients saw in that pain a gratuitous suffering. This highlights the importance of a good communication with the patient, and the involvement of the patient in the surgical process, as a way to reduce stress and improve pain.

In 1973 Marks and Sachar published a paper showing that numerous patients hospitalized for medical and surgical diseases suffered severe pain, had prescribed lower doses of analgesic than those accepted and also received doses much lower than prescribed. Unnecessary pain is described as pain that persist because of inadequate, insufficient or inexistent treatment. Clinical characteristics of postoperative pain make it perfect to treat adequately: It is predictable, its duration is limited, it does not fulfill any biological function, it appears in patients under strict control and frequently affects patients without important underlying diseases.

However, this same facility of treatment turns against him. His limited duration disregards health professionals and often makes patients themselves less demanding.

By definition, ERAS protocols assure patients the best evidence based care measures. In this chapter we analyze the influence of ERAS protocols in postoperative pain, and how this influence helps on reducing postoperative stay, postoperative complications and improving patients' experience of the surgical process, all of these proven results of the implementation of ERAS protocols.

Pain Control for Enhanced Recovery

Adequate Pain Control Is Key for ERAS Results

Enhanced Recovery after Surgery (ERAS) protocols have shown to reduce length of stay (LOS) and improve perioperative outcomes. Most studies have focused on colorectal surgery, but the success of ERAS programs has begun to translate to other surgical procedures as well. There are recent studies and meta-analyses that demonstrated the feasibility of ERAS implementation in bariatric surgery.

Post-operative analgesia requirements, post-operative nausea and vomiting, and impaired alimentation (a side from factors related to the operation) may drive prolonged LOS, and these may be amenable to operational improvement that benefits the healthcare system and patients by returning patients home sooner; therefore, optimal management of postoperative pain is an important component of ERAS protocols that can play a major role in how well patients recover after surgery. Inadequate pain management can prolong time to recovery milestones, such as mobilization and ambulation—lengthening hospital stays and leading to readmissions. Effective pain management can improve clinical outcomes and patient quality of life, while avoiding clinical complications, thereby saving healthcare resources.

Perioperative Analgesia

Postoperative pain is probably one of the worst treated kinds of acute pain, it can last hours and even days, it may condition patients attitude towards his own recovery and it has been classically overlooked for been considered normal.

Perioperative analgesia is the combination of measures that include managing pain in a preventive fashion, regular pain evaluation, efficient drug selection, perioperative rehabilitation and analgesic treatment for the outpatient. It has proven to improve patients' experience of the surgical process making them prone for an early discharge after surgery and reducing other pain induced postoperative complications.

The concept of perioperative analgesia started its evolution with the first anesthetics-based pain service to provide postoperative analgesia on surgical wards, which was first suggested over 30 years ago. This framework provided useful context for analysis that ultimately lead to the conclusion that the approach to managing surgical patient's pain should begin before the operation. It should involve pre-emptive analgesia, multimodal analgesia and perioperative rehabilitation. The physiologic basis and the techniques available for perioperative and multimodal analgesia have been discussed on previous chapters.

Perioperative analgesia is widely spread on *fast track* protocols and it has proven to have benefits that act as adjuvants on the enhanced recovery process, improving surgical quality. Some of these benefits are:

- Better pain control
- Reductions of opioids usage and dependence
- Earlier mobilization
- Reduction of nausea and vomiting
- Reduction of non-surgery related complications.
- Early accomplishment of discharge criteria.
- Improvement of patient experience.

One Result, Multiple Factors

Many of the items considered for fast track surgery have a direct or indirect impact on postoperative pain, from the preparatory consult where patients are made aware of what to expect and get involved as an active part of the process, to the surgical technique, anesthetic management, analgesia and drug selection, etc. As a result, the vast majority of publications that asses postoperative pain during the implementation of an ERAS protocol, in all kinds of surgery, report a significant difference when compared with pre-ERAS groups.

Multifactorial influence of ERAS protocols on postoperative pain is one of the conclusions of a recent meta-analysis from Chemali et al. While comparing 21 randomized controlled trials involving 1261 patients, they failed to find differences between analgesic procedures in the context of fast track protocols. When discussing these results, they noted that the most likely explanation is that standard ERAS protocols have multiple elements that may have a cumulative benefit on pain relief in addition to analgesic interventions which makes extremely difficult to assess the specific effect of the latter.

CONCLUSION

Postoperative analgesia has come a long way, but it is still far from perfection. ERAS protocols, based on evidence for best medical practice, have shown improvements in most postoperative outcomes including pain, with an approach that better understands its biological basis, but also adding to pharmacological analgesia, the implicit benefits of less invasive techniques, a consideration of patient's perspective of the surgical process and clear postoperative pathways. The tendency to improve results by implementing ERAS suggests that standardization of best proven strategies might be the key towards painless interventions.

Table 1. Data on postoperative pain of studies evaluating ERAS outcomes

Surgery	Author /Year	Country	N (ERAS/ nonERAS)	Variable	Results (ERAS/nonERAS)
Bariatric	King et al./ 2018	USA	715/366	Opioid consumption*	16.2 vs 41 ($p < 0.001$)
Bariatric	Ruiz-Tovar et al. /2018	Spain	233/286	Visual analogic scale	16 ± 12 vs 20 ± 28 ($p = 0.032$)
Colorectal	Liu et al. /2017	USA	3768/5556	Opioid consumption*	30.6 vs 52.4 ($p < 0.01$)
Orthopedics	Liu et al. /2017	USA	5002/1523	Opioid consumption* Mean acceptable pain score	27 vs 38.9 ($p < 0.01$) 72.7 vs 68.2 ($p < 0.01$)
Colorectal	Sarin et al. /2016	USA	279/245	Numerical pain score (0-10) 1st postoperative day 2nd postoperative day	 2.1 vs 3.2 ($p < 0.001$) 2.6 vs 3.2 ($p = 0.0019$)
Gynecology	Modesitt/ 2016	USA	136/211 249/324	Postoperative pain scores Opioid consumption*	3.7 vs 5 ($p < 0.01$) 15 vs 23.6 ($p < 0.01$)
Bariatric	Monika /2015	Poland	146/228	Visual analogic scale	2.4 vs 2.6 ($p=0.145$)
Orthopedics	Christellis /2015	Australia	297/412	Visual analogic scale: First 24 hours Rest Movement First 48 hours Rest Movement	 4 vs 5 ($p < 0.001$) 5 vs 6 ($p < 0.001$) 3 vs 4 ($p < 0.001$) 5 vs 6 ($p < 0.001$)

* Morphine equivalents (mg).

References

Baños Díez JE, Bosch-Llonch F, Farré Albaladejo M. *Historia de la terapéutica analgésica.* [*History of analgesic therapy*] Madrid, Ergon, 2006.

Bugada D, Bellini V, Fanelli A, et al. Future Perspectives of ERAS: A Narrative Review on the New Applications of an Established Approach. *Surg Res Pract* 2016: 3561249. https://doi.org/10.1155/2016/3561249.

Chemali ME, Eslick GD. A Meta-Analysis: Postoperative Pain Management in Colorectal Surgical Patients and the Effects on Length of Stay in an Enhanced Recovery after Surgery (ERAS) Setting. *Clin J Pain* 2017; 33 (1): 87–92.

Christelis N, Wallace S, Sage CE, et al. An Enhanced Recovery after Surgery Program for Hip and Knee Arthroplasty. *Med J Australia 2015;* 202 (7): 363–68.

King AB, Spann MD, Jablonski O, et al. An Enhanced Recovery Program for Bariatric Surgical Patients Significantly Reduces Perioperative Opioid Consumption and Postoperative Nausea. *Surg Obes Relat Dis 2018*. https://doi.org/10.1016/j.soard.2018.02.010.

Liu VX, Rosas E, Hwang J, et al. Enhanced Recovery after Surgery Program Implementation in 2 Surgical Populations in an Integrated Health Care Delivery System. *JAMA Surg 2017;* 152 (7): e171032.

Modesitt SC, Sarosiek BM, Trowbridge ER, et al. Enhanced Recovery Implementation in Major Gynecologic Surgeries: Effect of Care Standardization. *Obstetrics & Gynecology 2016;* 128 (3): 457–66.

Proczko M, Kaska L, Twardowski P, Stepaniak P. Implementing Enhanced Recovery after Bariatric Surgery Protocol: A Retrospective Study. *J Anesth 2016;* 30 (1): 170–73.

Ruiz-Tovar J, Muñoz JL, Royo P, et al. Implementation of the Spanish ERAS Program in Bariatric Surgery. *Minim Invas Ther 2018.* https://doi.org/10.1080/13645706.2018.1446988.

Sarin A, Litonius ES, Naidu R, et al. Successful Implementation of an Enhanced Recovery after Surgery Program Shortens Length of Stay and Improves Postoperative Pain, and Bowel and Bladder Function after Colorectal Surgery. *BMC Anesthesiol 2016;* 16 (1): 55.

Tan M, Siu-Chun Law L, Gan TJ. Optimizing Pain Management to Facilitate Enhanced Recovery After Surgery Pathways. *Can J Anesth* 2015*;* 62 (2): 203–18.

In: Management of Postoperative Pain ... ISBN: 978-1-53614-284-6
Editor: Jaime Ruiz-Tovar

Chapter 12

Single Port Approach and Influence of Placement of the Ports on Postoperative Pain

Andrés García Marín[1,*]***, MD, PhD***
and Mercedes Pérez López[2]
[1]Department of Pathology and Surgery,
University Miguel Hernández, Elche, Spain
[2]Department of Nursery, Hospital Universitario San Juan,
Alicante, Spain

Abstract

Single-incision laparoscopic surgery presents potential benefits over conventional approach such as a better cosmesis and less postoperative pain because of the reduction of abdominal wall trauma, with similar results in terms of operative time, complication rate, excess of weight loss and resolution of comorbidities. However, there is a little evidence to recommend it as a standard procedure. We have reviewed studies comparing the single-port versus multi-port approaches related to postoperative pain.

---

* Corresponding Author Email: andres.garciam@goumh.umh.es.

Keywords: pain, visual analogue scale, bariatric surgery, single-incision laparoscopic surgery

Introduction

Laparoscopic approach is the gold standard for bariatric surgery with many advantages over the open approach, such as less postoperative complications (wound infection and incisional hernia), pain, shorter length of hospital stay, faster recovery and better cosmesis [1].

Single-incision laparoscopic surgery (SILS) was described in 1992 but the first reports in bariatric surgery (adjustable gastric banding [AGB] and sleeve gastrectomy [SG]) appeared in 2008. The advantages over conventional laparoscopic approach are better cosmesis, potential for less postoperative pain due to fewer trocars and, therefore, reduction of abdominal wall trauma with less probability of bleeding and hematoma formation, since SILS also avoids the lateral placement of the ports and the risk of epigastric vessel injury, local nerve irritation, shorter length of hospital stay and development of incisional hernia. However, there is insufficient evidence to recommend SILS in the place of conventional laparoscopic approach.

Randomized controlled trials are needed to analyze the benefits of this technique [2-6].

A summary of the studies related to postoperative pain comparing single-port versus multi-port approach is presented below:

a) Saber et al. conducted a retrospective study comparing 14 SILS versus 12 conventional multi-port laparoscopic SG. They found a significant difference in postoperative pain score, measured by visual analogue scale (VAS), 4 versus 6.5 ($p = 0.003$) and a reduced need for opioid analgesia (71.4% versus 91.6%). The limitations of the study include the nonrandomized, retrospective nature, short follow-up time and the small sample size [4, 7].

b) Raman et al. conducted a retrospective study comparing 24 SILS versus 24 five multi-port AGB. They described significant differences in the mean period of postoperative painkillers use between SILS (2 days) and conventional group (5 days) [8].

c) Chakravartty et al. conducted a prospective study comparing 111 SILS versus 99 multi-port AGB. Operative time and complications rate were similar in both groups. Postoperative use for analgesia was significantly less in SILS group [9].

d) Rogula et al. conducted a nonrandomized study comparing 28 prospective SILS (14 SG and 14 Roux-en-Y gastric bypass) versus 28 conventional multi-port laparoscopic (14 SG and 14 Roux-en-Y gastric bypass) in patients with body mass index (BMI) $< 50kg/m^2$. Operative time, length of hospital stay, complications rate and excess weight loss (EWL) at 1 and 4 months were similar in both groups. VAS score was significantly higher on the first (SILS 5.0 ± 2.1, multi-port 6.5 ± 1.8, $p = 0.007$) and second (SILS 4.0 ± 2.0, multi-port 5.1 ± 2.4, $p = 0.049$) postoperative days in multi-port approach but the frequency of patient-controlled analgesia use and oral painkillers in hospital and after discharge were similar in both groups. Moreover, patients satisfaction was high in SILS group because of the vertical scar was well-hidden in the umbilical area [1].

e) Park et al. conducted a prospective nonrandomized study comparing 106 SILS versus 100 multi-port AGB. They reported that SILS patients presented significantly less pain at first ($p = 0.012$), twelfth ($p = 0.017$) and twenty-fourth postoperative hour ($p = 0.012$) as well as less need for oral painkillers ($p = 0.012$). No significant differences were seen in duration of patient-controlled analgesia use and parenteral narcotic consumption [10].

f) Lakdawala et al. conducted a prospective study comparing 300 SILS versus 300 conventional multi-port laparoscopic SG in patients with BMI $< 60kg/m^2$. EWL at 6 months, 1 and 2 years, the resolution of comorbidities and complications rate were comparable in both groups. They described that the postoperative need for painkillers between 4 and 8 hours was 30% of the SILS patients and 76% of the multi-port approach ($p < 0.0001$) and the need for painkillers on discharge was 0% versus 24% ($p < 0.0001$) respectively. The main limitation was the nonrandomized nature [7, 11].

g) Porta et al. conducted a randomized study comparing 65 SILS versus 65 conventional multi-port laparoscopic SG in patients with BMI < 50kg/m^2. Operative time, complications rate, EWL for the first four years and quality of life according to short form-36 were similar in both groups. They described similar mean and range VAS score on days 1 (2.1 [0-7] single-port, 2.0 [0-6] multi-port, $p = 0.46$) to 3 (0.6 [0-4] single-port, 0.7 [0-5] multi-port, $p = 0.90$) and postoperative paracetamol consumption in both groups [12].

h) Morales-Conde et al. conducted a randomized study comparing 15 SILS versus 15 conventional multi-port laparoscopic SG in patients with BMI<50 kg/m^2. Operative time, complications and EWL at 6 months were similar in both groups. Mean VAS score was significantly higher on the first (SILS 34.1 ± 8.9, multi-port 49.3 ± 12.2, $p = 0.046$) and second postoperative (SILS 22.1 ± 7.9, multi-port 35.9 ± 10.2, $p = 0.044$) days in multi-port approach but not on the third day [13].

Conclusion

In conclusion, SILS has showed similar results in terms of operative time, complications rate, EWL and resolution of comorbidities, with less use of postoperative analgesia and better cosmesis compared to multi-port approach. However, more randomized studies are previously needed to recommend it as a standard bariatric procedure.

References

[1] Rogula, T., Daigle, C., Dua, M., Shimizu, H., Davis, J., Lavryk, O., et al. Laparoscopic Bariatric Surgery Can Be Performed Through a

Single Incision: A Comparative Study. *Obes. Surg.,* 2014; 24: 1102 - 8.

[2] Dapri, G., El Mourad, H., Mathonet, P., Delaporte, A., Himpens, J., Cadière, G. B., et al. Single-Access Laparoscopic Adjustable Gastric Band Removal: Technique and Initial Experience. *Obes. Surg.,* 2013; 23:272 - 6.

[3] Reavis, K. M., Hinojosa, M. W., Smith, B. R., Nguyen, N. T. Single-laparoscopic incision transabdominal surgery sleeve gastrectomy. *Obes. Surg.,* 2008; 18:1492 - 4.

[4] Saber, A. A., Elgamal, M. H., Itawi, E. A., Rao, A. J. Single incision laparoscopic sleeve gastrectomy (SILS): a novel technique. *Obes. Surg.*, 2008; 18:1338 - 42.

[5] Nguyen, N. T., Hinojosa, M. W., Smith, B. R., Reavis, K. M. Single laparoscopic incision transabdominal (SLIT) surgery-adjustable gastric banding: a novel minimally invasive surgical approach. *Obes. Surg.*, 2008; 18:1628 - 31.

[6] Dimitrokallis, N., Alexandrou, A., Schizas, D., Angelou, A., Pikoulis, E., Liakakos, T. Single-incision laparoscopic sleeve gastrectomy: review and a critical appraisal. *J. Laparoendosc. Adv. Surg. Tech. A.,* 2017; 27:217 - 26.

[7] Lo, C., Latin, L., Fariñas, A., Cruz, C., Postoev, A., Ibikunle, C., et al. Does single-port laparoscopic sleeve gastrectomy result in improved short-term perioperative outcomes compared to conventional multi-port laparoscopic sleeve gastrectomy?. *Int. J. Surg.*, 2015;. 22:67 - 71.

[8] Raman, S. R., Franco, D., Holover, S., Garber, S. Does transumbilical single incision laparoscopic adjustable gastric banding result in decreased pain medicine use? A case-matched study. *Surg. Obes. Relat. Dis.*, 2011; 7:129 - 33.

[9] Chakravartty, S., Murgatroyd, B., Ashton, D., Patel, A. Single and multiple incision laparoscopic adjustable gastric banding: a matched comparison. *Obes. Surg.,* 2012; 22:1695 - 700.

[10] Park, K., Afthinos, J. N., Razi, S. S., Chan, E., Lee, D. Y., Teixeira, J. A. Laparoendoscopic single-site surgery for the placement of an

adjustable gastric band: a large cohort comparison. *Surg. Obes. Relat. Dis.,* 2013; 9:686 - 91.

[11] Lakdawala, M., Agarwal, A., Dhar, S., Dhulla, N., Remedios, C., Bhasker, A. G. Single-incision sleeve gastrectomy versus laparoscopic sleeve gastrectomy. A 2-year comparative analysis of 600 patients. *Obes. Surg.,* 2015; 25:607 - 14.

[12] Porta, A., Aiolfi, A., Musolino, C., Antonini, I., Zappa, M. A. Prospective comparison and quality of life for single-incision and conventional laparoscopic sleeve gastrectomy in a series of morbidly obese patients. *Obes. Surg.,* 2017; 27:681 - 7.

[13] Morales-Conde, S., Del Agua, I. A., Moreno, A. B., Macías, M. S. Postoperative pain after conventional laparoscopic versus single-port sleeve gastrectomy: a prospective, randomized, controlled pilot study. *Surg. Obes. Relat. Dis.*, 2017; 13:608 - 13.

In: Management of Postoperative Pain … ISBN: 978-1-53614-284-6
Editor: Jaime Ruiz-Tovar

Chapter 13

Importance of Nurse Management on Postoperative Pain

Covadonga Martín Garrido
Nursing Department,
Universidad Pontificia de Comillas, Madrid, Spain

Abstract

This chapter summarizes the job developed by a nurse to treat postoperative pain, especially focused on bariatric patients. Evaluation, classification and treatment of pain is considered. Finally, a care plan applicable to any patient undergoing bariatric surgery is developed.

Keywords: obesity, post-surgical pain, nursing, care plan

Introduction

Obesity is considered a disease that increases the risk of suffering other pathologies. The causes of obesity are very varied: genetic factor, abuse of fast-food, sedentary life-style, stress and socio-economic conditions. In addition, obesity implies an aesthetic problem with its corresponding psychological repercussion and diminishes the capacity to develop the normal activities. Body Mass Index (BMI) is the main parameter used to determine the obesity degree [1].

Obesity is so prevalent among the population in developed countries, that it is considered a public health disease. The World Health Organization (WHO) has named iy "the epidemy of the 21st century". Therefore, it is essential that the professionals, involved in the management of obesity, know the related risks, in order to treat the problems in an integral manner to take the appropriate solutions [2].

Bariatric surgery is the best alternative to treat morbid obesity, once dietary counselling, life-style changes and medical treatments have failed. The participation of nursing professionals is important, because it encompasses assistance, educational and nutritional aspects. Nurses are essential part of the multidisciplinary team, that will carry out this surgical intervention. The nurse works with the patient in a personalized and individualized way.

Nursing work with respect to the patient undergoing bariatric surgery is differentiated into three phases:

- Prior to surgery: the patient is cited with nursing to develop a specific initial assessment of vital signs, anthropometric parameters, personal medical history and allergies, as well as an exhaustive assessment of the feeding pattern, physical activity and self-image. The objective of this interview is to detect factors that may influence the outcome of bariatric surgery, as well as to determine the health education that the patient will need and to establish a relationship of trust [1].
- Admission phase: nursing addresses all the care techniques, including the emotional state and promoting the adaptation of the patient to the new situation that will help to improve the quality of life. Before being discharge, the nurse will prepare a report with the corresponding instructions and prescriptions for food, physical exercise, medication and upcoming revisions [1].

- After hospital discharge: nursing staff will monitor the evolution of the patient, assessing anthropometric and emotional aspects [1].

DEFINITION, CLASSIFICATION AND TREATMENT OF PAIN

Definition of Pain

Pain is a multidimensional experience that covers different aspects: physiological, sensorial, affective, cognitive, behavioral and sociocultural. The pain is unpleasant for the person who suffers it and is usually associated with a tissue injury. The perception of pain is due to the action of nociceptors (sensitive neuronal system) that can be modulated by other factors, such as psychological aspects [3].

The pain can cause physiological signs, such as high blood pressure, tachycardia, sweating and crying. It can also cause behavioral symptoms, like facial expression and anti-algic postures [3].

It is important to emphasize the direct treatment that nurses maintain with the patient and therefore the importance of all the nursing staff being able to identify, assess and treat pain accordingly.

Poorly controlled pain increases morbidity and mortality. Therefore, it is so important to detect and control it. Pain may cause other consequences in the patient, such as anxiety, insomnia, disorientation, agitation and delirium. In addition, poorly controlled pain can lead to chronicity and a depressive state. Thus, in patients with high levels of pain, the combination of analgesics and sedatives is used [4].

Classification of Pain

Pain can be classified according to its characteristics: origin, duration, cause, course, intensity and prognosis.

The origin of the pain can be very varied, since it can come from the disease itself, from an invasive procedure, from care techniques (placement of catheters and probes, aspiration of secretions, cures, mobilizations ...), of some infection and of the own immobility [4].

Through the prognosis, it is classified as difficult or complex pain to one that does not respond to the analgesia scale established by WHO.

To assess the pain three steps must be followed:

1. To get subjective patient information
2. To observe the behavior of the patient
3. To use measurement instruments (pain assessment scales)

Table 1. Classification of pain

Feature of pain	Types of pain
According to the duration	Acute: limited duration with little psychological impact Chronic: duration greater than 3 months, accompanied by the psychological component
According to the cause	Neuropathic: injury of nerve pathways or direct stimulation of the central nervous system Psychologic: the psychological and social sphere of the individual intervenes Nociceptive: local affection of the nervous terminal branches Somatic: localized pain that expands according to nerve paths Visceral: it does not have a clearly located focus and it can radiate to corporal areas far from its origin
According to the course	Continuous: does not disappear Irruptive: exacerbation of a stable base pain. Breakthrough pain is treated by the prevention and use of appropriate medication.
According to the intensity	Mild: does not interfere with usual activities Moderate: interferes with usual activities. It is treated with weak or minor opioids Severe: interferes with the rest. It is treated with major opioids

Table 2. WHO analgesic steps

Step I	Non-opioid analgesics + Coanalgesics (Paracetamol, NSAIDs, Metamizole)
Step II	Minor Opioids (Codeine, Tramadol) + Coanalgesics + Step I
Step III	Major Opioids (Morphine, Oxycodone, Fentanyl, Methadone) + Coanalgesics + Step I
Step IV	Invasive + Coanalgesic methods.

The WHO analgesic scale establishes the order of use of analgesics, allowing to control pain adequately in over 80% of cases.

To correctly apply this scale, it is important to determine the intensity of the pain and to correctly monitor it. It must climb step when the previous one fails. The pattern of coanalgesics depends on the cause of the pain and should be maintained even if you step up. The combination of minor and major opioids is not appropriate. It is important that there is a pattern of analgesia that covers the breakthrough pain in case it appears.

Pain Assessment and Monitoring

Pain is a subjective experience and therefore it is necessary to interview the patient. The nurse will determine the value of pain, combining what is stated by the patient along with what can be assessed objectively [4].

Painful perception can be modified by various situations, such as previous painful experiences, age, emotional state and cognitive state [4].

The ideal is to assess the pain by quantification using specific scales. These scales should be used every 4 hours, always respecting the patient's diet and rest [4].

There are several scales to assess pain. If the patient has communication skills, the Visual Analogic Scale (VAS) can be used, but if the patient is not able to communicate, the Campbell scale is indicated [4].

In addition to assessing pain, the response to treatment must also be evaluated to determine whether it is effective or not [4].

VAS Scale (Visual Analogy Scale)

It consists of a line that shows the numbers from 0 to 10, representing 0 "absence of pain" and 10 "unbearable pain." The distance of the line separates the intensity of the pain. To use this scale it is necessary that the patient has good motor and visual function. It is not useful in sedated or elderly patients.

0	1	2	3	4	5	6	7	8	9	10

Figure 1: Visual Analogic Scale (VAS) ranging from 0 to 10

Graduation of pain:

- From 1 to 3: mild/moderate pain
- From 4 to 6: moderate/severe pain
- From 6 to 10: very intense pain

We must bear in mind that the same word may have different meanings for different patients.

VNS Scale (Verbal Numeric Scale)

Similar to the VAS scale, but in this case, the patient simply expresses, verbally or in writing, the value of pain ranging from 0 to 10, with 0 representing "absence of pain" and 10 "unbearable pain." This scale is very useful in critical patients.

Verbal Descriptive Scale

The patient classifies his pain around 6 defined degrees (no pain, mild pain, moderate, intense, very intense and unbearable).

No pain	Soft pain	Moderate pain	Intense pain	Very intense pain	Unbearable pain

Figure 2: Verbal descriptive scale

Campbell Scale

This scale assesses the presence of pain and quantifies its intensity, through the assessment of 5 items: facial muscles, tranquility, muscle tone, verbal response and comfort. It is used in patients unable to communicate. Its score range goes from 0 to 10, being ideal to keep the score below 3. 0 is considered no pain, from 1 to 3 is mild-moderate pain, from 4 to 6 is moderate-severe pain and above 6 very intense pain.

Table 3: Campbell scale

Indicator	**0**	**1**	**2**
Facial muscles	Relaxed	Tense, frown, grimace	Frown and clenched teeth
Tranquility	Relaxed, quiet, normal movements	Occasional movements due to restlessness	Frequent movements
Muscular tone	Normal	Increased (flexion of fingers)	Rigid
Verbal response	Normal	Complaints, crying, whining or occasional grunts	Complaints, crying and frequent grunting
Comfort	Comfortable, quiet	Calms to touch and/or voice, is easily distracted	Difficult to comfort through touch or voice

Wong-Baker scale

It was designed to assess pain in children. It shows faces with different facial expressions, associating happiness with absence of pain and increasingly sadder expressions as the intensity of the pain increases. In addition, it is also useful for evaluating pain in patients with an inability to describe or understand the assessment scales, such as illiterate people, patients with cognitive impairment and the elderly.

In case the patient is intubated with non-deep sedation, we can assess their pain by asking clearly about it, giving it the necessary time to respond. They usually can communicate with movements, so VAS or VNS scales are used.

When the patient is not able to communicate and/or is under deep sedation, nursing assesses pain through indirect tools.

Through the information of the relatives we can also obtain great information regarding the pain of the patient since they can estimate the absence or presence, being more difficult to detect the degree of intensity.

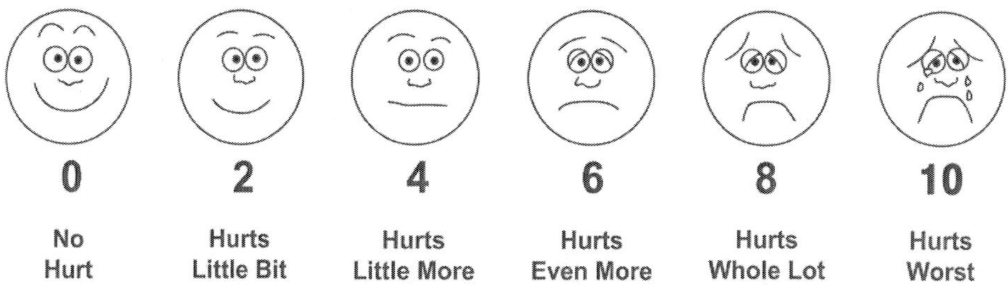
0
No Hurt
2
Hurts Little Bit
4
Hurts Little More
6
Hurts Even More
8
Hurts Whole Lot
10
Hurts Worst

Figure 3: Wong Baker scale

Postoperative Pain

Nurses work through direct contact with the patient, making it possible to assess and treat pain in a human way. Being able to recognize the suffering in the patient, convert nurses in humanized professionals in care. For this, nurses apply their own deontological code, based on protecting, maintaining and restoring the patient's health, as well as their autonomy, physical and mental functions, always individualizing for each patient.

The postoperative pain is due to the surgical procedure and is an acute pain, limited in time, predictable and therefore avoidable. Poor control of postoperative pain implies a negative impact on quality of life, functional recovery and increased risk of postoperative complications, morbidity and costs [5].

A good control of postoperative pain depends on the knowledge of the professionals and the experience they have [5].

During the postoperative period nursing staff applies care, trying to identify and treat early complications that may arise due to surgery or anesthesia, so that it offers quality care and safety. Among the postoperative aspects, one of the most important is the approach to pain.

Postoperative pain must be controlled because nurses have the knowledge and drugs necessary to treat it correctly. Appropriate control of pain supposes a good professional practice and great quality of care [5].

There are different drugs and administration routes useful to alleviate postoperative pain, and although there is the analgesia scale established by the WHO, in each country the policy of analgesia varies [5].

The treatment of postoperative pain should be preventive, that is, anticipate its appearance. Postoperative pain is suffered by more than 50% of patients undergoing surgery and increases complications by 15%. A correct control of postoperative pain decreases postoperative morbidity [5].

It must be borne in mind that each patient responds differently, and that the pain intensity after the same interventions might vary, depending on several factors. Therefore, the treatment must be individualized for each patient depending on the type of surgery [5].

It is important to take responsibility for the pain of others, considering their treatment as a fundamental human right. According to the Charter of Human Rights of the United Nations (year 2000) the treatment of pain is a universal right of human beings [5].

Standardized Care Plan for a Patient Undergoing Bariatric Surgery

As already explained throughout this chapter, obesity supposes an increased risk of suffering other pathologies, premature death, a reduction of up to 20 years of life and an associated socio-health cost.

Bariatric surgery is an alternative surgical treatment to address obesity. It is very important to establish an individualized and realistic care plan. An effective care plan must be valuated daily.

Table 4. Standardized Care Plan: Provision to improve health management

Diagnosis	Provision to improve health management
Definition	Pattern of regulation and integration in the daily life of a therapeutic regimen for the treatment of the disease and its sequelae, which can be reinforced
NOC	Compliance behavior: prescribed diet Definition: personal actions to follow the intake of fluids and foods recommended by a health professional for a specific health disorder Indicators: 1. Select foods and liquids compatible with the prescribed diet. 2. Select rations compatible with the prescribed diet. 3. Drink liquids compatible with the prescribed diet. 4. Follow the recommendations to organize the diet.
	Knowledge: pain management Definition: degree of knowledge transmitted on the causes, symptoms and treatment of pain. Indicators: 1. Causes and factors that contribute to pain. 2. Signs and symptoms of pain. 3. Strategies to control pain 4. Importance of following the medication regimen.
NIC	Improvement of self-confidence Definition: strengthen a person's confidence in their ability to perform healthy behavior. Activities: 1. Explore the individual's perception of their ability to develop the desired behavior. 2. Explore the individual's perception of the benefits of executing the desired behavior. 3. Help the individual to commit to an action plan to change behavior. 4. Provide positive reinforcement and emotional support during the learning process and during the implementation of the behavior.
	Empowerment of self-esteem Definition: help a patient to improve the personal judgment of their self-worth. Activities: 1. Encourage the patient to identify their strengths. 2. Refrain from negative criticism. 3. Help establish realistic goals to achieve higher self-esteem. 4. Encourage the patient to accept new challenges.

Table 5. Standardized Care Plan: Obesity

Diagnosis	**Obesity**
Definition	Problem in which an individual accumulates an abnormal or excessive level of fat for their age and sex, which exceeds the levels of overweight
NOC	Weight loss behaviour Definition: personal actions to lose weight with diet, exercise and behavior modification Indicators: - Select a healthy target weight. - Controls the food ration. - Controls body weight. - Controls the body mass index.
	Management control of eating disorder Definition: degree of knowledge transmitted about an eating disorder, its treatment and the prevention of the progression of the disease and complications. Indicators: 1. Healthy target weight. 2. Healthy nutritional practices. 3. Strategies to promote satisfaction with body image. 4. Strategies to prevent relapse.
NIC	Nutritional advice Definition: use of an interactive help process focused on the need to modify the diet. Activities: - Establish a therapeutic relationship based on trust and respect. - Discuss the meaning of the food for the patient. - Value the efforts made to achieve the objectives.
	Set limits Definition: establish the parameters of a desirable and acceptable behavior of the patient. Activities: - Indicate, limit or identify (with the participation of the patient, as appropriate) the undesirable behavior of the patient. - Establish the consequences (with the participation of the patient, when appropriate) of appearance/absence of desired behaviors. - Avoid discussing or negotiating the consequences and behavioral expectations established with the patient. - Use a constant, practical, non-judgmental method. - Communicate the limit in positive terms

Table 6. Standardized Care Plan: Risk for electrolyte imbalance

Diagnosis	**Risk of electrolyte imbalance**
Definition	Vulnerable to changes in serum electrolyte levels, which can compromise health
NOC	Electrolytic balance Definition: concentration of the serum ions necessary to maintain the balance between the electrolytes.
NIC	Electrolyte monitoring Definition: collection and analysis of patient data to regulate electrolyte balance. Activities: 1. Monitor the serum level of electrolytes. 2. Identify possible causes of electrolyte imbalances. Recognize and notify about the presence of electrolyte imbalances. 3. Consult the doctor if the signs and symptoms of imbalance of fluid and/or electrolytes persist or worsen.

Table 7. Standardized Care Plan: Anxiety

Diagnosis	**Anxiety**
Definition	Vague feeling of threat or discomfort, accompanied by autonomous response, caused by the anticipation of a danger.
	Related factors: lack of information on hospitalization, surgical experience and therapeutic regimen at discharge.
	Defining characteristics: restlessness, uncertainty, confusion, worry, pulse increase.
NOC	Control of anxiety: actions to eliminate or reduce feelings of apprehension and tension from an unidentifiable source. Indicators: 1. Look for information to reduce anxiety 2. Refers absence of physical manifestations of anxiety
NIC	Decrease anxiety: minimize apprehension, fear, omen related to the source of unidentified danger and in advance. Activities: 1. Presentation of the staff to the patient and family 2. Explanation of all procedures 3. Provide objective information on the diagnosis and treatment

Table 8. Standardized Care Plan: Risk of deterioration of sleep pattern

Diagnosis	Risk of deterioration of sleep pattern
Definition	Long periods of time without periodic suspension, naturally sustained by relative unconsciousness. Related factors: change in the usual sleep and wake schedules, anxiety, interruptions for therapeutic procedures, noise, lighting, pain.
NOC	Sleep: magnitude and pattern of periodic suspension of consciousness during which the body recovers. Indicators: 1. Quality of sleep 2. Hours of sleep
NIC	Environmental management: comfort. Manipulation of the environment to facilitate optimal comfort. Activities: 1. Position the patient in a way that facilitates body alignment 2. Avoid unnecessary interruptions, grouping care and allowing rest 3. Adjust the room temperature 4. Determine irritating environmental factors
	Promotion of sleep: facilitate regular sleep and wakefulness cycles. Activities: 1. Determine the patient's sleep pattern 2. Observe and record the number of hours of sleep 3. Explain the importance of adequate sleep for proper recovery 4. Explain to the family the appropriate visiting hours

Table 9. Standardized Care Plan: Self-care deficit–food, hygiene and elimination

Diagnosis	Self-care deficit: food, hygiene and elimination
Definition	Impairment of the person's ability to perform or complete the described activities on their own. Related factors: postoperative rest, therapeutic devices Defining characteristics: immobility, fear, pain
NOC	Personal care: activities of daily life. Ability to perform the basic tasks of personal care. Indicators: 1. Food 2. Hygiene 3. Use of the toilet

Table 9. (Continued)

Diagnosis	Self-care deficit: food, hygiene and elimination
NIC	Help with self-care: food. Help eat. Activities: 1. Place the patient in a comfortable position 2. Provide pain relief 3. Explain the preparation of special diets
	Help with self-care: bathing and hygiene. Activities: 1. Provide the necessary privacy for grooming 2. Provide or prepare the necessary material 3. Monitor the condition of the skin 4. Maintain oral hygiene
	Help with self-care: cleanliness. Activities: 1. Encourage the patient to ask for help 2. Help with the use of the potty or wedge 3. Ensure the necessary privacy

Table 10. Standardized Care Plan: Degradation of physic mobility

Diagnosis	Degradation of physic mobility
Definition	Limitation of independent movement Related factors: prescription of postoperative restriction of movements, discomfort or pain, overweight, therapeutic devices Defining characteristics: immobilization, resistance to the change of position, cuffed by fear and pain
NOC	Mobility level. Ability to move with resolution. Indicators: 1. Maintenance of body position 2. Maintenance of balance 3. Ambulation
	Safety behavior: prevention of falls. Actions to minimize the risk factors that could cause falls. Indicators: 1. Correct use of help device 2. Use of containments if necessary 3. Provision of personal assistance
NIC	Teaching of the activity and prescribed exercise. Prepare the patient to achieve the prescribed activity level.

Diagnosis	Degradation of physic mobility
NIC	Activities: 1. Inform the patient of the purpose and benefits of the exercise 2. Report appropriate activities according to their physical condition 3. Warn of the dangers 4. Explain the importance of early ambulation to avoid the formation of thrombi
	Ambulation. Activities: 1. Encourage wandering when your physical situation allows 2. Provide physical or mechanical assistance needed to walk 3. Schedule walks according to physical condition
	Prevention of falls. Establish special precautions in patients at high risk of injury from falls. Activities: 1. Control gait, balance and fatigue when walking 2. Provide support and support devices

Table 11. Standardized Care Plan: Risk of deterioration of skin integrity

Diagnosis	Risk of deterioration of skin integrity
Definition	Risk of skin being negatively affected Related factors: humidity, mechanical factors, immobility, overweight and secretions.
NOC	Tissue integrity: structure and normal physiological function of the skin and mucous membranes. Indicators: 1. Intact skin 2. Absence of tissue damage
	Risk control. Actions to eliminate or reduce health threats. Indicators: 1. Recognizes the possible health risks 2. Recognize changes in health status
NIC	Care of the bedridden patient. Promote comfort, safety and prevention of complications in the patient who cannot get out of bed. Activities: 1. Position the patient appropriately 2. Keep the bedding clean and dry 3. Encourage the patient to make passive movements

Table 11. (Continued)

Diagnosis	Risk of deterioration of skin integrity
	Surveillance of the skin. Activities: 1. Observe if there is reddening or loss of skin integrity per turn 2. Monitor humidity and temperature 3. Monitor the correct placement of devices in contact with the skin and mucous membranes 4. Maintain scrupulous hygiene
	Prevention of pressure ulcers. Activities: 1. Daily skin monitoring, especially in risk areas 2. Cleaning and hydration after bathing 3. Placement of protectors 4. Schedule postural changes 5. Observe if there are sources of excessive pressure or friction

Table 12. Standardized Care Plan: Poor knowledge regarding food

Diagnosis	Poor knowledge regarding food
Definition	Lack or deficiency of cognitive information related to a correct diet. Defining characteristics: ignorance about healthy dietary habits Related factors: overweight, uncontrolled intake, composition and caloric value of food
NOC	Knowledge: diet. Degree of understanding issued on diet. Indicators: 1. Description of the recommended diet 2. Explanation of the relationship between diet, exercise and weight 3. Description of the allowed meals 4. Meals to be avoided
	Weight control. Personal actions to achieve and maintain an optimal body weight for health. Indicators: 1. Maintains a recommended dietary pattern 2. Seek professional help when you need it

Diagnosis	Poor knowledge regarding food
NIC	Stages in the oral diet. Insist on the necessary restrictions of the diet with the consequent progression of it according to tolerance. Activities: 1. Establish diet progressively 2. Observe and record tolerance to the progression of the diet 3. Instruct on how to prepare dietary supplements
	Teaching: prescribed diet. Activities: 1. Explain the purpose of the diet 2. Provide a written meal plan 3. Teach how to select the right foods 4. Explain the importance of diet 5. Plan exercise and activities 6. Weight control weekly
	Nutrition monitoring. Data collection to avoid or minimize malnutrition. Activities: 1. Observe the skin 2. Monitor the occurrence of nausea or vomiting 3. Control by blood analysis 4. Weigh the patient at the established intervals 5. Observe the existence of diarrhea

Table 12. Standardized care plan for acute pain management

Diagnosis	Acute pain
Definition	Unpleasant emotional and sensory experience caused by a real or potential tissue injury or described in such terms; sudden or slow onset of any intensity from mild to severe with an anticipated or foreseeable end of a duration of less than six months.
NIC	Pain management. Activities: 1. Pain assessment: type, location, beginning of pain 2. Observe non-verbal indicators of discomfort 3. Use pain control measures 4. Mediate before an activity to increase participation 5. Evaluate pain control measures regularly
	Analgesic administration. Activities: 1. Checking the prescription of analgesia 2. Checking the history of allergies 3. Administration of the drug at the dose, time and established route 4. Record of the analgesic response and any adverse effects

REFERENCES

[1] Rodríguez Alonso J, Plaza del Pino FJ, Puentes Sánchez J. [Bariatric surgery and integral nursing attention]. *Biblioteca Lascasas,* 2006; 2:3.

[2] Del Pino Salgado M, Ayestaran Guillerna I, Ferrero Mozo MT, Jiménez Mendía MD. [Risks perception for the safety of the patient assesseded by the professionals involved in the process of bariatric surgery from admission to ICU discharge].*URPA 2016;3:1.*

[3] Puebla Díaz F. [Types of pain and WHO therapeutic scale: Iatrogenic pain. *Oncología (Barcelona)* 2005;28(3):33-37.

[4] Pardo C, Muñoz T, Chamorro C. [Pain monitoring. Recommendations from the Analgesia and Sedation Task Force from the SEMICYUC]. *Med Intensiva* 2006;30(8):379-385.

[5] Sagastume JR. [*Postoperative pain: Where are we going?*] Sirena: Poesia, arte y critica 2005:2-3.

ABOUT THE EDITOR

Jaime Ruiz-Tovar, MD, PhD is General and Digestive Surgeon, specialized in Bariatric Surgery. He works actually in the Center of Excellence for the Treatment of Obesity in Valladolid (Spain). He is also the Academic Director of Surgery at the University Hospital Rey Juan Carlos and is the Head of Obesity Department at Garcilaso Clinic, both in Madrid (Spain). His teaching career is actually developed at two universities; he is Associated Professor of Surgery at the Universidad Autonoma de Madrid and is Associated Professor of Health Sciences at Universidad Alfonso X. He is the Coordinator of the Bariatric Section in the ERAS-Spain group and has coauthored the new Guidelines for Bariatric Surgery, endorsed by the Spanish Surgical Association (AEC) and the Spanish Society for Surgery of Obesity (SECO). His research interests are focused on bariatric surgery and surgical infection.

INDEX

A

B

C

D

E

F

P

Q

R

S

T

U

V

W